Praise for
Man Up! A Practical Guide
for Men in Nursing

"This book is the definitive volume on men in nursing and describes how to position them to become nurses, to assume leadership positions, to seek and receive mentoring, and to make a difference in the workforce. It provides a historical context, describes barriers, and recommends strategies for the future. This volume should be required reading for faculty, deans, and CNOs as well as any courses on professionalism and leadership. Guidance counselors and admission officers, who tend to steer men and women away from the nursing profession, should also read this. While the lived experience of Chris Coleman and of the chapter authors enriches each chapter, the history of data and the practical recommendations make the book a reader-friendly classic. This book will be a milestone and a turning point for balancing gender in schools of nursing and the health workforce."

–Afaf I. Meleis, PhD, DrPS (hon), FAAN
Margaret Bond Simon Dean of Nursing
Professor of Nursing and Sociology
University of Pennsylvania School of Nursing

"The appalling lack of diversity in our profession continues to fuel our contentment with the status quo and lack of forward momentum. Christopher Coleman and colleagues enter this critical dialog with pragmatic support for men who are considering or currently navigating a career in nursing. The first-hand narratives will assist many men in finding their voice within our profession and provide all a deep understanding of the richness that comes with diversity."

–F. Patrick Robinson, PhD, RN, ACRN
Dean, Curriculum and Instruction
Chamberlain College of Nursing

"I am pleased to endorse *Man Up!* Christopher Coleman and Sigma Theta Tau International have taken a strong position for the profession to become more friendly to men and more gender-diverse. The authors accurately describe the current state and provide the context for doors to open wide for gender inclusion and balance in nursing. Reading *Man Up!* gave me a new sense of optimism and energy. I hope it does for you too."

–William T. Lecher, MS, MBA, RN, NE-BC
President, American Assembly for Men in Nursing
Senior Clinical Director, Cincinnati Children's Hospital Medical Center

"Drawing on experiences from both very accomplished men and emerging leaders, *Man Up!* provides first-hand advice for making the most of opportunities in nursing[md]from prelicensure student to leader, researcher, and entrepreneur. Its review of issues in promoting gender and other forms of diversity in nursing—and wealth of inspiring examples of career success from different generations—will find audiences and stimulate discussion across the profession."

–Sean Clarke, PhD, RN, FAAN
Professor, Susan E. French Chair in Nursing Research
Director, McGill Nursing Collaborative
Ingram School of Nursing, McGill University, Montreal

"*Man Up!* is a great read if you are a man thinking of entering the nursing profession. The chapter authors challenge readers to do their homework and acquire the kind of information needed to make smart choices on types of programs, locations, and available support. ManUp! creates a vision of nursing that is intellectually demanding and physically challenging. Nursing provides social connections and meaning and is well-respected and compensated—it's a great career choice."

–William L. Holzemer, PhD, RN, FAAN
Professor and Dean, College of Nursing
Rutgers, The State University of New Jersey

"This group of authors provides expert advice for all, but specifically men. The book is packed with critical knowledge and practical actions for those considering entering nursing, those in practice who are pondering future directions, and mentors of men in nursing. I gained many new insights from this volume as will all who read it."

–Thomas L. Hardie, EdD, RN, PMHCNS-BC, NP
Associate Professor of Nursing, Drexel University
Retired Full Professor, University of Delaware
Adjunct Full Professor, University of Pennsylvania

"Chris Coleman and his colleague authors expertly blend practical information with critical insights into today's world of nursing. They help readers envision where our profession is going and how to be a leader within it. He gives us an invaluable primer for success in practice and leadership."

–Kathleen M. McCauley, PhD, RN, ACNS-BC, FAAN, FAHA
Associate Dean for Academic Programs and Professor of Cardiovascular Nursing
University of Pennsylvania School of Nursing
Past President, American Association of Critical-Care Nurses

"*Man Up!* provides a powerful perspective on the special challenges of men working in the traditionally female-gendered nursing profession. The authors give readers a mix of practical advice and wise insights. This book should be read by all nurses—male and female. Ultimately, creating an inclusive and collaborative profession is key to the future of nursing. Christopher Coleman and colleagues have designed the blueprint to that future."

–Kathleen Dracup, PhD, RN, FNP, FAAN
Dean Emeritus, UCSF School of Nursing

Man Up!

A Practical Guide for Men in Nursing

Christopher Lance Coleman
PhD, MS, MPH, FAAN

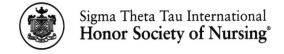

Sigma Theta Tau International
Honor Society of Nursing®

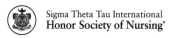

Sigma Theta Tau International
Honor Society of Nursing®

> The Honor Society of Nursing, Sigma Theta Tau International (STTI) is a nonprofit organization whose mission is to support the learning, knowledge, and professional development of nurses committed to making a difference in health worldwide. Founded in 1922, STTI has 130,000 members in 86 countries. Members include practicing nurses, instructors, researchers, policymakers, entrepreneurs and others. STTI's 482 chapters are located at 626 institutions of higher education throughout Australia, Botswana, Brazil, Canada, Colombia, Ghana, Hong Kong, Japan, Kenya, Malawi, Mexico, the Netherlands, Pakistan, Portugal, Singapore, South Africa, South Korea, Swaziland, Sweden, Taiwan, Tanzania, United Kingdom, United States, and Wales. More information about STTI can be found online at www.nursingsociety.org.

Sigma Theta Tau International
550 West North Street
Indianapolis, IN, USA 46202

To order additional books, buy in bulk, or order for corporate use, contact Nursing Knowledge International at 888.NKI.4YOU (888.654.4968/US and Canada) or +1.317.634.8171 (outside US and Canada).

To request a review copy for course adoption, e-mail solutions@nursingknowledge.org or call 888. NKI.4YOU (888.654.4968/US and Canada) or +1.317.634.8171 (outside US and Canada).

To request author information, or for speaker or other media requests, contact Rachael McLaughlin of the Honor Society of Nursing, Sigma Theta Tau International at 888.634.7575 (US and Canada) or +1.317.634.8171 (outside US and Canada).

ISBN: 9781937554873
EPUB ISBN: 9781937554880
PDF ISBN: 9781937554897
MOBI ISBN: 9781937554903

Library of Congress Cataloging-in-Publication Data

Man up! : a practical guide for men in nursing / [edited by] Christopher Lance Coleman.

  p. ; cm.

Includes bibliographical references.

ISBN 978-1-937554-87-3 (book : alk. paper) -- ISBN 978-1-937554-88-0 (EPUB) -- ISBN 978-1-937554-89-7 (PDF) -- ISBN 978-1-937554-90-3 (MOBI)

I. Coleman, Christopher Lance, 1962-

[DNLM: 1. Gender Identity. 2. Nurses, Male. 3. Nursing--organization & administration. WY 191]

RT41

610.73081--dc23

2013012492

First Printing, 2013

Publisher: Renee Wilmeth
Acquisitions Editor: Emily Hatch
Editorial Coordinator: Paula Jeffers
Cover Designer: Alan Berry
Interior Design/Page Layout: Katy Bodenmiller

Principal Book Editor: Carla Hall
Development and Project Editor: Kevin Kent
Copy Editor: Keith Cline
Proofreaders: Michelle Melani, Andrew Kimmel
Indexer: Johnna Van Hoose Dinse

Dedication

I dedicate this book to my late grandmother Mary Bell Sterling who taught me the meaning of courage, and who epitomized what it meant to break up "unhealthy traditions." When I entered our noble profession, I encountered "unhealthy traditions" that perpetuated the notion that men were to "stay in their place, and not be heard." While the profession has evolved in a positive direction with respect to diversity and equality, there still exist "institutionalized glass ceilings" that unfortunately continue to challenge men at every level in nursing. Like my grandmother, I believe in breaking up "unhealthy traditions" because they eventually hurt us all. Every contributor to this book has forged a path for men in nursing and for men who are considering pursuing the nursing profession. These are the men who asked for gender-neutral language in our textbooks and in our classrooms where the nurse is still referred to as "she." Not long ago, I was at a gathering where a prominent nurse leader was describing the ideal person for a leading position and kept using the pronoun *she* when describing the "ideal candidate." I do not believe this was intended; however, the choice of words is a byproduct of institutionalized thinking that inspired me to contribute this work. I want to inspire men, nursing deans, nursing students, and nurses at every level to strategically create measurable change and opportunities for men who aspire to lead our national organizations or to serve as deans or as chief nursing officers. Our diversity is our strength, and if we all commit to changing "unhealthy traditions" like my grandmother did, we will create equity that will bring tremendous opportunity to all who want to enter our noble profession.

Acknowledgments

I would like to express gratitude to the men who took time out of their very busy schedules to commit to contributing to this book. I am also grateful to Emily Hatch, Carla Hall, the entire publishing team, and the Sigma Theta Tau International Board of Directors for their commitment to this important contribution to nursing.

About the Author

Christopher Lance Coleman, PhD, MS, MPH, FAAN

Christopher Lance Coleman is the Fagin Term Associate Professor of Nursing and Multicultural Diversity and is Co-Director of the Center for Health Equity Research at the University of Pennsylvania School of Nursing. He received his BS from Walla Walla University, his MS from Oregon Health Science University, and his PhD with a minor in education from the University of California, San Francisco. Additionally, he completed a post-doctoral fellowship at UCLA and earned an MPH from the Johns Hopkins University School of Public Health.

He holds memberships in numerous organizations such as the Honor Society of Nursing, Sigma Theta Tau International and the American Academy of Nursing. Additionally, he serves on multiple editorial boards and is a peer reviewer for a number of refereed journals. He has published research articles and book chapters, has received federal funding from the National Institutes of Health (NIH) and intramural funding for HIV/AIDS, and completed a study in Botswana. He was a mayoral appointee to the Ryan White Title-I Planning Council for the City of Philadelphia and served on the board of directors for the Association of Nurses in AIDS Care and the National Association on HIV Over Fifty.

Additionally he served as Vice Chair and Interim Chair of the Community Advisory Board, Center for AIDS Research, University of Pennsylvania, and served as chairman of the board of directors for HAVEN Youth Center Inc 1997–2013. He has made both television and radio appearances discussing HIV/AIDS in the Black community. His research focuses on health disparities, particularly on understanding the numerous factors that influence health-promoting behaviors of HIV-infected middle-aged African-American men and HIV and STD risk factors among vulnerable populations who may be incarcerated, homeless, or mentally ill and he has a particular interest in the role of spirituality and religion on physical and mental health.

In 2007, he was elected to the American Academy of Nursing for his outstanding scientific contributions. His published book, *Dangerous Intimacy: Ten African American Men with HIV*, featured on Amazon.com, is the result of his work with seropositive African-American men.

Contributing Authors

Jeffrey L. Bevan, MSN, RN, FNP-BC, CEN

Jeffrey L. Bevan is a nationally board-certified family nurse practitioner and currently serves as an assistant professor and nurse practitioner program coordinator for Mount Carmel College of Nursing in Columbus, Ohio. Prior to entering the nursing profession, Bevan started out in EMS as a paramedic. He completed his bachelor of science in nursing degree at Ohio University in Athens, Ohio, and his Master of Science in Nursing degree at Otterbein University in Westerville, Ohio. He is currently working towards a research doctorate in nursing at Rush University in Chicago, Illinois. With over 20 years of experience in the health care field, Bevan utilizes his diverse background in nursing to enhance his academic role. In addition, he continues to provide direct care for patients as an FNP in a large asthma, allergy, and immunology practice in Central Ohio.

Kevin Daugherty Hook, MA, MSN, CRNP

Kevin Daugherty Hook, chief nursing officer, University of Pennsylvania, LIFE program, is a nurse practitioner with extensive clinical experience in CCU/ICU settings as clinician and preceptor. He has experience in program development, leadership, and education in long-term care and national professional organizations. Hook has been a recipient of awards for patient care.

Paul J. Larson, MS, RN

Paul J. Larson is clinical academic coordinator at Gundersen Lutheran Medical Center, La Crosse, Wisconsin, and adjunct faculty with the University of Wisconsin-Madison School of Nursing. He teaches junior and senior nursing students at the Western Campus of the University of Wisconsin-Madison School of Nursing (at Gundersen Lutheran Medical Center), and local high school students in the La Crosse School District's Health Academy. He is Gundersen Lutheran's site coordinator for the National Database of Nursing Quality Indicators (NDNQI), and president of the local chapter of the American Assembly for Men in Nursing. He received his master's degree in Community Health Education from the University of Wisconsin-La Crosse and his bachelor's degree in nursing from Viterbo University.

Jonathan Lee, BS, RN

Jonathan Lee is a recent graduate of the UCLA School of Nursing. While at UCLA, he co-founded Men in Nursing at UCLA and was the organization's president until his graduation. Under his leadership, the group was quickly recognized as an official chapter of the American Assembly for Men in Nursing and became one of the largest and most active chapters of the assembly. As an individual and through the American Assembly for Men in Nursing, he continues to challenge the stereotypes and inequalities that affect all nurses and hold back the nursing profession. Lee is also a member of Sigma Theta Tau International.

Brent MacWilliams, PhD, ANP

Brent MacWilliams is an assistant professor, University of Wisconsin-Oshkosh, ACCEL Leadership: Research and Evaluation, and member of the Board of Directors, American Assembly for Men in Nursing. He is an adult nurse practitioner with a nursing background in the acute care setting. Brent holds a PhD in Education with a focus on online curricula design. He is a member of the Accelerated Leadership Team with responsibilities for Research and Evaluation. MacWilliams has been on the board of directors for American Assembly for Men in Nursing and Wisconsin Center for Nursing. As the principle researcher in a community-based partnership with Fort HealthCare, he won the National Perinatal Association-Model of Care for 2012, which focused on prevention of shaken baby syndrome.

Steven A. Marks, MS, RN

Steven A. Marks, operations manager, Clinical Skills and Simulation Center, Mount Carmel Health. The center is designed to be used by medical students, medical residents, the nursing school, staff nurses and allied health professionals, paramedics, and even organizers of community training sessions such as for those caring for a relative at home. The center includes both hospital room settings and a mock apartment with living room, bedroom, kitchen, and bathroom and also can be used by programs such as therapy for disabled veterans re-learning daily tasks.

Daniel J. Pesut, PhD, RN, PMHCNS-BC, FAAN, ACC

Daniel J. Pesut, past president of the Honor Society of Nursing, Sigma Theta Tau International, is professor of nursing, Population Health and Systems Cooperative Unit and the Katherine R. and C. Walton Lillehei Chair in Nursing Leadership at the University of Minnesota School of Nursing. He is also director of the Katharine J. Densford International Center for Nursing Leadership.

Franklin Shaffer, EdD, RN, FAAN

Franklin Shaffer, chief executive officer, CGFNS International was previously executive vice president of Cross Country Healthcare and chief nursing officer for Cross Country Staffing. He was appointed by the Joint Commission on Accreditation of Healthcare Organizations (JCAHO or the Joint Commission) to serve on their Nursing Advisory Council. Prior to his tenure with Cross Country Staffing, Shaffer served as chief nursing officer at several medical centers, deputy director for the National League for Nursing and adjunct faculty in graduate nursing programs at Teachers College, Columbia University; Adelphi University; and Hunter College.

Steven Simpkins, RN

Steven Simpkins has had a long-term career in hospitality and customer service before he discovered his interest in nursing. He received his bachelor of nursing science in 2010 from the University of Washington and immediately after graduation was admitted to the PhD program in the School of Nursing at the University of Washington. He is currently a Graduate Assistance in Areas of National Need Scholar focused on nursing education. As a GAANN Fellow he has completed multiple teaching and research fellowships. He is in his third year of his PhD training, having completed certificates in HIV and Sexually Transmitted Diseases and in Nursing Education. Simpkins will take his general exams and advance towards candidacy in the summer of 2013. His service activities are extensive and include treasurer of Sigma Theta Tau International, Psi-at-Large chapter and the Association of Nurses in AIDS Care, Puget Sound Chapter, and committee chair of fundraising for the Northwest chapter of the National Gerontological Nurses Association.

Roy L. Simpson, DNP, RN, DPNAP, FAAN

Roy L. Simpson is vice president, nursing informatics, at Cerner Corporation. As such, he is responsible for strategic sales and relationships for the patient care enterprise, as well as representation at the industry level for Cerner's nurse practice. Simpson has more than 30 years of experience in nursing informatics and executive administration. His primary executive research focus pioneered the development and funding of the Nursing Minimum Data Set (NMDS). The NMDS is a minimum set of nursing data elements with uniform definitions and categories, including nursing problems, diagnoses, interventions, and patient outcomes approved by the American Nurses Association

Spencer Barrington Stubbs

Spencer Barrington Stubbs, BSN candidate 2013, is president of the Male Association of Nursing at the University of Pennsylvania, president of the Onyx Senior Honor Society, and an elected student body representative for the entire undergraduate nursing school body. Spencer is also active in other nursing school groups on campus through his participation as an executive board leader to both the Minorities in Nursing Organization (MNO) and the Penn Understanding Sexuality in Healthcare (PUSH). Stubbs is also a participant in the Ronald E. McNair Scholars program and the Mellon Mays Undergraduate Fellowship program.

Joachim G. Voss, PhD, RN, ACRN

Joachim G. Voss is an Associate Professor in the Biobehavioral Nursing and Health Systems Department in the University of Washington School of Nursing. Voss was a Fulbright Fellow in 1998/99. He has focused on HIV-related symptom management of fatigue and the identification of biomarkers for fatigue since 2000. He pioneered the development of the first mitochondrial oligonucleotide gene expression microarray during his time as research fellow at the NIH. Voss has been funded as a principal investigator since 2003 from the NIH, the University of Washington, and recently by the Robert Wood Johnson Foundation.

Table of Contents

Foreword

When I was growing up in Washington, DC, during the 1960s, change was constantly in the air: civil rights marches, the poor people's campaign, peace demonstrations, Earth Day, the moon landing. In the middle of this, my parents had a long-ago friend from England come into town. He mentioned that he was a nurse, and the day went on with no sense of scrutiny. A male nurse—okay. Good to know.

A few years later, I worked in Virginia at what was a Boy Scout reservation—six camps around a lake surrounded by national forests. A large staff provided programs to thousands of Scouts. Being on staff, I would go to the central dispensary. The fellow in charge impressed me, as he ran a tight but caring operation. I was a liberal arts major in college, and my direction was unsure. This fellow seemed like a good person to ask for advice. He was a nurse working on his doctorate. He told me that nursing was a career that could provide a sense of purpose, security, and variety. I applied to prenursing science courses and started within a month.

Nursing school and eventually nursing practice come with challenges for men. Stereotypes about gender roles come from different directions—neighbors, friends, teachers, classmates of both genders. Comments and questions come in all varieties:

- It's great to have men in nursing.

- Can men really be as caring as women in taking care of suffering patients?

- Where is your hat?

- Do men have an unfair advantage in rising to the top when historically, nursing has been one of the few professions where women could hold high positions?

- How does it feel to be a *male* nurse (as if being a male nurse were different than being a nurse)?

Interestingly, such curiosity was rare when I was providing care. Work at the bedside and as a teacher was exactly what that fellow in Virginia had promised—I had a sense of purpose, security, and variety.

Man Up! A Practical Guide for Men in Nursing provides in-depth perspectives for men considering or already going into nursing. The lead author, Christopher Lance Coleman, has brought together a group of men from a variety of leadership roles in nursing. In this volume, they provide insights and articulate issues in a thoughtful, comprehensive, and powerful way. Becoming a leader, shaping the profession, and making a difference are all the more real with the strategies they describe for becoming an effective clinician, administrator, professor, or researcher, or a combination of those roles. Their advice resonates for me as I mentor students and faculty. This book is an important contribution toward advancing the nursing profession.

I was honored to be a speaker at the American Assembly for Men in Nursing (AAMN) meeting this year in San Francisco. As I looked out on the audience, I saw a sea of men, all committed to excellence in nursing. Each was networking, sharing information, and thinking about how to improve care or the preparation of caregivers. The number of men considering and going into nursing is increasing. Each of us has had an inspiration. For me, the fellow from England, the man in Virginia—these nurses provided a vision that has given me a sense of purpose, security, and variety. This volume provides inspiration and, more than that, practical advice on becoming successful as a nurse leader.

David Vlahov, PhD, RN, FAAN
Dean and Professor
School of Nursing
University of California, San Francisco

Introduction

"Knowledge will bring you the opportunity to make a difference."

— *Claire M. Fagin, PhD, RN, FAAN*

I am pleased to welcome you to *Man Up! A Practical Guide for Men in Nursing*. The goal of the book is to provide you strategies for navigating through the nursing profession. I have assembled nursing students and nurses in clinical practice, administration, and academia to give you their perspective about how to achieve your goals and objectives in the nursing profession. Each chapter will present a formula for succeeding in a female-dominated profession. Whether you are a student or a nurse on the frontlines, their pragmatic advice will capture your imagination and inspire you with wisdom that will enable you to join the ranks of men making history.

Did you know that according to statistics from the American Association of Colleges of Nursing (AACN) men comprise just 7% of U.S. registered nurses and only 5% of nursing faculty teaching from the baccalaureate to the PhD? Further, only 4.5% of school of nursing deans are men (2012). These statistics not only underscore the gender disparity, but also present an opportunity for men to enter a profession with reasonable job security and a decent salary. In 2010 the Institute of Medicine (IOM) challenged the nursing profession to diversify its workforce by gender as well as to consider the larger implication of recruiting men to reduce the nationwide nursing shortage.

A pragmatic solution would be to populate schools of nursing around the country with men in leadership roles in the academic and in the practice arena. Seeing more men in a female-dominated profession has the potential for changing the landscape of nursing on a larger scale. I believe men need a guide, a blueprint to use to navigate through the complexity of specialty choice and a culture where frankly a gender disparity still exists. This is an opportunity of a lifetime for men to not only change the face of nursing in the 21st century, but also to reshape the public image that nursing is a women's profession. As David Vlahov, PhD, RN, FAAN, dean of the UCSF school of nursing stated, "Nursing is not a woman's profession, it is a people's profession" ("Men Slowly Change the Face of Nursing Education," 2012).

Man Up! A Practical Guide for Men in Nursing has the potential, through nationwide and international-wide dissemination, to shake up the status quo by educating men using real-world dialect and common-sense wisdom. This guide provides a roadmap that will enhance the likelihood of a successful career in clinical, academic, or administrative tracks in nursing.

For too long we have lacked a practical guide for men choosing nursing or who are in the nursing profession to use as a pragmatic resource. One of my heroes, Dr. Claire M. Fagin, the first woman to serve as chief executive officer of the University of Pennsylvania and the first woman to serve a term as interim president of any Ivy League university is quoted as saying, "Knowledge will bring you the opportunity to make a difference." Presently, she is Leadership Professor Emerita and Dean Emerita at Penn. Dr. Fagin used her knowledge to blaze trails to leadership for nurses all over the world. Dr. Fagin has truly inspired me to employ strategic actions to make a difference. Like Dr. Fagin, I recognize imparting knowledge is the pathway to change no matter how complex the challenges one may experience. *Man Up! A Practical Guide for Men in Nursing* delivers our primary objective to impart knowledge to students, clinicians, academicians, and those in administration, so that we can make a difference in the status quo of nursing.

The book is divided into three parts. The first part (Chapters 1 through 4) discusses approaches for successfully navigating through nursing school, gender communication, and strategies for carving out your presence. The second part (Chapters 5 through 7) focuses on a framework for mentorship, lack of racial diversity and innovative ways to diversify the nursing workforce. The final part of the book focuses on useful approaches for developing leadership skills, as well as the importance of engaging in your organization, and gives you a blow-by-blow account of what it is like to be male student in a nursing program. In short, *Man Up! A Practical Guide for Men in Nursing* provides a roadmap for men in nursing, schools of nursing, and hospitals looking for guidance to enhance their environments.

My goal is that this guide offers you practical approaches to effectively crafting a successful career in nursing. I want you to come away with tangible strategies that can be used if you are a student, a professor, or an administrator that will enable you to reach your goals and objectives. I believe that presenting you with the voices of successful male nursing leaders as well as students gives this guide a level of credibility you will not find in any other text. This is what makes the book a must read for every male considering nursing, men who are currently in the nursing profession striving towards advancement, hospital administrators seeking to diversify their workplace, and for deans seeking to recruit male students and faculty. Like Dr. Fagin, I believe imparting knowledge does and can make a difference; my ultimate goal is for *Man Up! A Practical Guide for Men in Nursing* to make a measureable difference for nursing nationally and internationally.

References

American Association of Colleges of Nursing (AACN). (2012). Retrieved from http://www.aacn.nche.edu/research-data/ standard-data-reports

Men slowly change the face of nursing education. (2012). Robert Wood Johnson Foundation. Retrieved from http://www.rwjf. org/en/about-rwjf/newsroom/newsroom-content/2012/04/men-slowly-change-the-face-of-nursing-education.html

Chapter 1

So You Want to Become a Nurse

Christopher Lance Coleman, PhD, MS, MPH, FAAN
Fagin Term Associate Professor of Nursing
University of Pennsylvania School of Nursing

If you're a man considering going into nursing, prepare yourself. The statistics are against you. Men currently comprise only 6.6% of the nursing workforce. Wait, it gets worse. Want to work in an academic setting? In the academic arena, men represent only 5% of full-time faculty and just 4.5% of the nursing deans, according to the latest statistics released by the American Association of Colleges of Nursing (AACN, 2012). Though daunting, this gender gap provides a tremendous opportunity for men considering a career in nursing and looking to diversify the profession. What you learn in this chapter will help you navigate the various pathways to becoming a nurse.

Inform Yourself Before Talking with Your Parents

As a male, one of many challenges you face when considering nursing is to educate those around you about why this noble profession is right for you (Bartfay, Bartfay, Clow, & Wu, 2010). Families often expect their sons to choose traditional male-dominated fields such as medicine, dentistry, or law. For example, although I considered these careers paths, the universe had a different trajectory for me; my father was disappointed about this and remained silent about my choice to pursue nursing.

Some of the challenging conversations that took place between my family and me involved explaining to them the events that influenced my decision to pursue nursing. During those robust discussions, I found it helpful to share a significant example about an emergency room nurse who managed a complex trauma case with grace, strength, and leadership. I shared how witnessing this nurse in action represented the "tipping point" for me. Looking back on those conversations, I now clearly see that, at the core, my family (and the public in general) perceived nursing as a woman's profession (Harding, 2007; Neilson & McNally, 2012; Roth & Coleman, 2008). My parents worried that a man choosing nursing would face obstacles such as stigma, limited opportunities, and low pay, to name a few. The word *bedpan* kept creeping into conversations. Eventually, though, my family acquiesced, thinking that I would eventually change my mind.

So, how should you prepare yourself for this conversation? First, educate yourself about the facts; be prepared to inform your parents about all of the different opportunities available to nurses, such as research, teaching, and the variety of clinical areas. Also, they must learn about the different roles nurses have within these areas. You need to have key talking points in mind when you speak to your parents: nurses can move just about anywhere to work, you can support your family on the salary, you will have tremendous opportunity for advancement, the numbers of men who are nurses is growing, men can serve in leadership roles, the technology is amazing, and most importantly, you will have job security.

WHAT YOUR PARENTS MIGHT SAY	WHAT YOU CAN SAY
Female profession	Leadership opportunities
Changing bedpans all day	Job security
Money not good	Great salary
No profession for a man	Movability
Taking doctors' orders all day	Advancement opportunities

Take Your High School Sciences Courses Seriously

After you've explained your plans to your family, what do you need to consider next? Easy. You need to know how to ensure a smooth and ultimately successful nursing school application process. While you are still in high school (and most states do require a high school diploma for licensure), do well in your classes, especially biology, chemistry, psychology, mathematics, and physics. Nursing programs evaluate academic achievement in the sciences and prefer above-average performance as an indication of the likelihood of successful progression through a program.

Get Work Experience

Although you want to get good grades, a nursing school admission's committee evaluates more than just grades; they consider your work experience relevant. For example, individuals who have worked as a Certified Nursing Assistant (CNA) have an advantage because of their clinical exposure to nurses and the fact that they have provided direct basic patient care. This work experience also demonstrates a serious commitment to the field of health care, and specifically to an applicant's commitment to pursuing a career in nursing.

In addition, if educational financing presents an issue for you, working as a CNA could be a gateway into basic or vocational nursing, such as the Licensed Practical Nurse. Although this role has career-advancement limitations, it provides an opportunity to perform basic patient care and administer medications, which would provide great entry-level experience toward the Registered Nurse (RN) licensure, which in most cases opens the door to completion of a bachelor's degree and higher.

Applying to Nursing School

At this point, you will no doubt ask, "How do I get into nursing school? How do I submit the best application?" Earlier, I mentioned the high school prerequisites. Now I want to share some suggestions to ensure that your application stands out from the crowd:

- **Be sure that your application sparkles.** The application is your only voice during the admissions committee deliberations. So, check for typos and be neat.

- **Accept help.** Have others review your writing and consider their suggestions.

- **Brag about your accomplishments.** This is not the time to be shy. List all your accomplishments, including awards, student leadership, club and organization memberships, and volunteer activities. You need to present a well-rounded representation of your academic experience.

- **Seek strong academic recommendations.**

- **Volunteer in a health care setting.**

- **Student leadership will make you look strong.**
- **Join nursing organizations.** Students usually get a discounted rate.
- **Visit the school.** And do your homework.

Choosing Which Degree to Pursue

The beauty of nursing is the variety of degree options. For example, you might opt to enroll in a 3-year program or a bachelor's degree. Beyond the undergraduate degree await the master's and doctoral degrees. Learn about which degrees your potential employers require before you enroll in any program. Specifically, investigate whether they prefer the bachelor's degree for employment versus a 3-year degree.

DIFFERENCES BETWEEN 4- AND 3-YEAR NURSING PROGRAMS

BSN (4-Year)

- *Entry to leadership*
- *Exposed to nursing research and health policy*
- *Entry to MSN and PhD*
- *Becoming a requirement for employment at top-tier hospitals*
- *Longer duration, but fantastic investment*

ASN (3-Year)

- *Entry to clinical practice*
- *Not sufficient for advanced degrees*
- *Little exposure to nursing research or policy*
- *Shorter duration, but not a good long-term investment*

> **NOTE**
>
> *If you plan to work in a hospital, consider that most hospitals today prefer a nurse to hold a bachelor's degree.*

As another important part of your homework, research all the options schools offer. Some programs offer the traditional 4-year plan of study, a registered nurse – bachelor of science in nursing [RN-BSN]) program, or an accelerated program for those who hold degrees in other fields of study. You can choose a path that heads toward a successful career as a health care professional or one that takes you toward academia or research. In essence, the dynamic nursing profession offers many pathways. Other possible combinations with a BSN are a master of public health (MPH), master of business administration (MBA), PhD, or a juris doctor (JD) law degree, for example. The opportunities are limitless.

Research the Schools

Now you need to do your research about the school. Inquire about the National Council Licensure Examination (NCLEX) passage rate over the past 5 years. The gold standard is 90% or better, but check your state board of nursing to determine *their* metric for nursing schools.

Consider Ethnic Diversity

Ask about student ethnic diversity. Being the only ethnically diverse student at a school can be challenging. It can be a lonely experience not seeing anyone who looks like you or being at a school that does not value ethnic diversity. I was the only African-American male in all of my courses, from BSN to PhD, and that was challenging, because I felt at times I was dealing with perceptions that were not accurate. I highly recommend looking at schools that have diversity and inclusivity in their strategic plan. Also, inquire about student groups because these can be a wonderful support through school.

How Male Friendly Is the School?

You also want to determine the gender diversity of the school. For example, ask about the number of male faculty and of male students enrolled. Don't be shy. After all, you're considering a quite significant financial and personal commitment.

The answers to these important questions about ethic and gender diversity will allow you to make an informed decision about where to apply.

Other questions to consider asking include the following:

- How many students commute versus those that reside on campus?
- Has the school been recognized for diversity?
- What is the ethnic makeup of the student body?
- Do their published brochures reflect diversity?
- How flexible is the curriculum?
- Can I combine my nursing degree with another degree from another school?

Pay a Visit

Finally, visit the campus; do not just rely on literature to impress you. During your visit, you will get a feel for the atmosphere and culture of the school, and this should enlighten your decision-making process. I would recommend the following checklist for your visit:

- Ask to meet with current students, male and female.
- Ask the male students to share their experience.
- Meet with the student leaders.

- Meet with the faculty.
- Take a tour of the facilities, labs, and classrooms.
- Take a tour of the campus.

Prepare Yourself for the Courses

Now, imagine for a moment that the school has accepted you as a student. Now what? Well, you can expect to enroll in nursing courses intended to prepare you for clinical work. Each program has different iterations, but with fairly universal basics. Required courses during your 4 years will likely include a mixture of sciences, nursing fundamentals, pathophysiology, and clinicals. Table 1.1 shows what the courses look like over a typical 4-year nursing program.

TABLE 1.1 Typical 4-Year Nursing Degree Courses

FIRST YEAR	SECOND YEAR
Anatomy and physiology	Nursing clinicals
Biology	Anatomy and physiology II
Microbiology	Women and children
Liberal arts course requirements	Pathophysiology
Chemistry	Pharmacology
Human development	Liberal arts requirements
THIRD YEAR	**FOURTH YEAR**
Nursing clinicals	Community health nursing
Pediatrics	Nursing research
Mental health	Nursing leadership
Ethics	Liberal arts requirements
Adult and older adult health	Nursing clinicals
Statistics	

Note that this table merely presents an example of a typical nursing program and is in no way representative of all programs. Your opportunities in nursing are limitless.

Take Clinicals Seriously

As you can see from Table 1.1, where they appear in 3 of the 4 years of this particular nursing program, nursing clinicals represent an important component of nursing education. During these clinicals, you build the necessary skills to deliver competent nursing care.

Clinicals are hands-on and skill-building experiences through which you learn much about nursing care, including how to do the following:

- Properly make a bed
- Administer medications
- Listen to lung and abdominal sounds
- Conduct pharmacology quizzes
- Insert a Foley catheter, IV, and feeding tubes
- Perform range-of-motion exercises

Clinicals also expose you to clinical simulation of real-world medical events and all the innovative technology used in the hospitals. For instance, most hospitals have converted to electronic medical records, so expect training in this area.

The clinical training involves both developing laboratory skills and providing care to the patient at the bedside. Your instructors will expect you to integrate the theoretical content, the simulation lab experience, and the bedside care.

Commit Yourself to Excellence

Yes, all of this might seem overwhelming, but two crucial survival tips can help you navigate the rigors of a nursing program: First, believe in yourself and commit to giving it your all. Second, persist.

Having taught clinicals for many years, I know that most of my students would say that clinicals resemble internships or residencies required of most medical students. During clinicals, you have the opportunity to experience a variety of specialties: pediatrics, maternity, geriatrics, medical surgical care, mental health, acute care, chronic care, and so on. In addition, you have the opportunity to spend time in the community either providing home care or working in an extended-care facility or outpatient clinic.

As a student, you must show specific skill proficiencies before entering the hospital or care setting. Most schools, for example, require that students demonstrate competency in administration of medications, dosage calculations, procedures such as inserting a Foley catheter, IV administration, dressing changes, and so on before the school will approve them for clinical experiences.

So what does "giving your all, or committing to excellence" look like?

- **Immerse yourself in the readings**—Not just those required, but outside readings as well.

- **Improve your weaknesses**—If note-taking is not your thing, learn how to take good notes.

- **Attend all classes**—This is critical to a successful clinical experience

- **Ask your instructor for different experiences**— The more you do the more you will learn.

- **Do not just pick the easy-to-care-for patients**— Pick those with complex medical problems; this will enhance your critical-thinking skills.

Be Persistent

As you progress through each year of school, the skill complexity increases and becomes more intense, so persistence is the second key to survival.

The clinical experience provides the school an opportunity to evaluate whether students have achieved competency in skills learned in simulation and the classroom. The school and the medical community are not looking for robots; they're looking for skilled clinicians who can think critically while dealing with the medical complexity inherent in clinical settings. In addition, this is when you are developing professionalism and showing leadership. Students often ask, "What are clinical instructors looking for?" Well, it's not just their evaluation that is important; the floor RN's perception of you matters, too!

Be inquisitive. Ask to participate in any experience where you have the opportunity to learn new skills. Some of my students have shared that picking patients with complex medical needs enabled them to really learn how to think like a nurse (both an art and a science) and to learn incredible skills. 86toronado (2011), an emergency department RN, also recommends spending time preparing your clinical, letting the nurses know you are interested in learning everything possible, checking your school policy about what students are allowed and not allowed to do, having your care plans completed, and helping your fellow students.

Stay Focused in School

Finally, you must survive nursing school. So, attend all classes. Focus in class—ask questions, pay attention, and take notes. Because of the intensity of nursing, students must assimilate an enormous amount of material, so forming a study group is prudent. With the explosion of technology and social media, you might discover classmates spending time on social media outlets during class. Avoid this pitfall and discipline yourself to fully focus on learning. Live a balanced life, exercise, eat a healthful diet, and get plenty of sleep. Get to know your professors, and make office appointments.

Doing the readings before class is essential. And because of the sheer volume of required reading, you will find that highlighting important take-home messages from the lectures is critical to your success.

Forster (2008) identifies mistakes to avoid while in nursing school that you may find quite helpful. First, she suggests that you research the career or specialty path you intend to pursue. For example, spend time in a variety of specialty areas so that you can investigate your interest in working within different areas.

Forster also recommends that you not just jump into any program. Instead, she suggests that you link your program to your career path. If you seek a higher degree, have a plan that takes you there. For instance, if you know that you do not intend to spend your entire career working on the floor but are instead seriously considering a PhD as a long-term goal, carefully plan with the program the trajectory of your career goals. Consult with your nursing program administration about how best to achieve your objectives.

As Forster also suggests, be mindful of changing programs in the middle of your education. Given the expense and investment required for nursing school, you must carefully consider whether your courses would even transfer to another institution.

Finally, Forster insists that you recognize the significance of embarking on a career in nursing and really appreciate the time demands and intensity of navigating through the coursework and clinicals. Nursing is demanding, and striking a balance between the demands of nursing and life outside of nursing is crucial.

> **NOTE**
>
> *To augment Forster's advice, I want to encourage you to take advantage of the available resources at colleges or universities, such as student psychological services and the academic support office. It is easy to forget the rich resources available to you through your program. Because no one is immune to stress, you want to have a support system that provides the structure and reinforcement necessary to ensure a successful journey.*

After you complete the program, you must sit for the NCLEX-RN exam before you begin your career as a professional nurse. At that point, review books/courses can help you to prepare; choose whatever works best for you.

In this chapter you have been provided with a pathway to nursing. You have much to consider as you prepare for this academic challenge. I have discussed the importance of preparation through education. The most difficult part for most men is convincing their families and some friends that choosing nursing is a viable career for a man. Before you can do this, you need to gather facts about the variety of positions in which nurses are employed. You also need to consider your entry point into nursing (ASN vs. BSN) and the differences between them. Think hard about your best pathway to leadership as you consider the best entry point. With the strategies for surviving the gender preconceptions, the academic rigor, and the clinical aspects you have learned in this chapter and will learn in this book, you can prepare yourself to succeed.

MEN IN NURSING SURVIVAL TIPS

Be prepared before talking to your family about your career plans.

Take your schooling seriously.

Research the best school for your interests.

Visit the campus and the faculty to learn about the student body and the resources.

Don't just rely on brochures and pamphlets as you consider schools.

Consider gender and ethnic diversity in your decision-making.

Find out about the school's NCLEX passage rates and history of accreditation.

Consider how visible the nursing school is on campus.

Have short-term and long-term goals.

Build a cast of supporting individuals around you.

References

American Association of Colleges of Nursing (AACN). (2012). Retrieved from http://www.aacn.nche.edu/research-data/standard-data-reports

Bartfay, W. J., Bartfay, E., Clow, K. A., & Wu, T. (2010). Attitudes towards men in nursing education. *The Internet Journal of Allied Health Sciences and Practice, 8*(2), 1-7.

86toronado. (2011). How to survive and thrive in nursing schools. Retrieved from http://allnurses.com/showthread.php?t=532725

Forster, H. (2008). 5 mistakes to avoid in your nursing education. Retrieved from http://nursinglink.monster.com/education/articles/4466

Harding, T. (2007). The construction of men who are nurses as gay. *Journal of Advanced Nursing, 60*(6), 636-644.

Neilson, G. R., & McNally, J. (2012). The negative influence of significant others on high academic school pupils' choice of nursing as a career. *Nursing Education Today*, doi:10.1016/j. nedt.2012.019

Roth, J. E., & Coleman, C. L. (2008). Perceived and real barriers for men entering nursing implications for gender diversity. *Journal of Cultural Diversity, 15*(3), 148-52.

Chapter 2

Stumbling into Leadership: Does Gender Matter?

Kevin Daugherty Hook, MA, MSN, CRNP
Adult and Gerontologic Nurse Practitioner, CNO
LIFE UPenn, University of Pennsylvania School of Nursing

Like many men, nursing was a second career for me (actually a third). My professional nursing career followed a stint as a high school English teacher, a graduate degree in religious studies and ethics, and a few years with a large entertainment corporation. I had long desired a career in nursing, but for many reasons had not pursued one. Shortly after I started work as a bedside nurse in the intensive care unit / critical care unit (ICU/CCU), a hospital chaplain remarked that what made older people coming into the nursing profession interesting was that our work identities were not "formed in the crucible of the hospital." Since then, I have pondered that remark and wondered in what ways nurses such as I might be doing things differently. Although I have several observations on this topic, the most germane to leadership is that those of us who came to nursing later and now find ourselves in leadership roles bring an outsider's view to nursing in general and to health care organizations in particular. To what degree this hinders or hampers our professionalization as nurses is another topic. I have concluded, however, that in terms of leadership, it is a good thing.

CONFRONTING THE HOSPITAL HIERARCHY

For instance, the historical hospital hierarchy, which many times gets in the way of patient care, was something I observed nearly immediately. I had actually assumed that in health care calling a physician so I could bring a concern forward would be met welcomingly. However, I learned early that this was not always the case and that a nurse's observations were not always received happily. Nor were they always believed. The top-down mentality was quite pervasive. I had worked in a corporate setting that welcomed different viewpoints; that was my professional norm. The hospital culture was an about face. I found this counterproductive, not to mention shocking, and would complain to unit management. I actually submitted a written complaint at one point against a physician whose behavior was totally inappropriate toward nursing staff. Was my reaction because I was a male? Because I came from a different work culture? Hard to discern, but I did notice that my female colleagues did not have the visceral responses I did about such behavior, at least not those women who had had no other work experience but hospital-based nursing. A number of studies performed have shown adverse patient outcomes as a direct result of how physicians behave towards nursing, including frequent studies showing a relationship between patient safety and physician-nurse relationships (Grena, P., & Lauve, R., 2006; Rosenstein, A., & O'Daniel, M., 2008; Saxton, R., Hines, T., & Maithe, E., 2009). So my observations have been validated.

My First Informal Steps Toward Leading in Nursing

My path to health care leadership started with my choice of undergraduate nursing program. I chose a fast-track post-baccalaureate, one that moved me through undergraduate nursing in a year and a half. Even in the undergraduate program, the expectation was that my entire cohort would head directly to our master's degrees as nurse practitioners, thereby taking on clinical leadership roles without much in the way of beside nursing experience. Either because of that program or because of my innate interests, most likely combinations of both, I immediately began looking for opportunities to connect with the larger nursing community to see where I could be of use and to broaden my fledgling nursing career. Ultimately, during my 7 years in hospital nursing, I joined a variety of nursing organizations, served on one work group, served as a board member on two others, and joined a few others to see what they might offer. In terms of my nursing colleagues on the unit, I found myself very much alone in these endeavors. Leadership on the unit, however, always encouraged my pursuits, and I began receiving hospital awards for my work (both at bedside and for extracurriculars).

I did not look ahead in any strategic way to formal leadership roles, something at odds with observations that men in leadership typically do (Moran, Duffield, Donoghue, Stasa, & Blay, 2011; Tracey & Nicholl, 2006). I did not look at work as a means to a particular end, again at odds with some observations (Tracey & Nicholl, 2006). My career goals were, to borrow from Tracey and Nicholl (2006), *diffuse*. At the time, my energy went to learning about and helping to work toward the larger nursing concerns at the widest professional level, in whatever form that took.

Forming and Recognizing My Leadership Style

During my nurse practitioner graduate education, my cohort again was exhorted to become leaders, with an overt focus on doing research and contributing to the nursing literature; in essence, get published. However, I did not go into direct clinical practice after finishing my nurse practitioner program. Instead, I began working for a large long-term care organization, reporting directly to the senior vice president (SVP) of clinical operations. In that role, I developed a nurse practitioner program, a new role for the organization. So, my graduate education definition of *leader* was not used, but I was most certainly leading. I did, however, find myself observing the senior vice president, her scope of influence, and how her role was shaped by the organization and how she, in turn, shaped her role. I became intrigued with formal leadership but gave little thought to next steps.

> **NOTE**
>
> *While I was certainly always looking forward to opportunities to expand my professional network and interests, I was unconscious about wanting a formal leadership role. No one looked like me or seemed to think the way that I did. I did not seek a mentor, nor did anyone come forward and speak to me about formal leadership.*

Part of the reason I was never approached about formal leadership, certainly during graduate school, was because I was focusing strictly on being an advanced clinician. The traditional graduate program for nurses who already know they want formal leadership is usually nursing administration or perhaps an MBA in health care administration. But it is certainly possible that because I was a man, people assumed if I wanted some leadership role, I would be going after it. I know many men who are in positions of leadership in nursing for whom it was clear early on that this was the path they wanted to take. It can be difficult to know where you want your nursing career to go. However, I suspect younger men coming into nursing already feel more comfortable in nursing, and thus, they are more comfortable about asking for what they want in terms of mentoring and information and will go get it. Is my falling into different roles without benefit of an active mentor attributable to my being a man for some reason? Perhaps a traditional male approach would have been more focused about going after one leadership role after another "to build a résumé" and more assertive about getting mentors on board to help. Or perhaps this is just an idiosyncrasy of my personality. I suspect a bit of both.

During these few years, I became aware that this was where my career would, or should, be going (although I never wanted to fully abandon my clinical expertise). So now I work for a hospice occasionally as an advanced practice nurse. I do so both because I like it and to keep my clinical skills somewhat intact, even as I am now at my third position, now with the title of chief nursing officer (CNO). This position came to me both through having maintained my relationships with faculty from graduate school and my colleagues from there.

The practice where I work is an ambulatory practice serving frail elders at the low end of the socioeconomic scale and historically clinically underserved. The practice is staffed primarily by nurse practitioners and nurses, but it is a truly interdisciplinary model, complete with physicians, social workers, recreation therapists, physical and occupation therapists, a clinical nutritionist, as well as Certified Nursing Assistants (CNAs). Despite my title of CNO, physical and occupational therapists report to me, and likely the CNAs will too in the near future. I work closely with the chief medical officer to ensure quality and best-evidence practice and direct nursing goals according to the Institute of Medicine's (IOM) report about ensuring organizations allow nurses at all levels practice to their full scope. And I work closely with the chief operating officer (COO) when our spheres of influence overlap.

My current role came to me as a result of graduate program connections and recommendations from colleagues from my school of nursing who knew my prior work. But, I was not looking, nor did I particularly seek, a position with the title CNO. In that sense, I am aware that I have actually stumbled onto a high-level leadership role. After more than a year in the role now, I understand that given my clinical and management history I am at a point that requires a more conscious and active assessment of my career goals as well as my leadership skills and weaknesses.

Paradoxically, nursing was the career I chose following a period in the corporate world, where a sense of accomplishment through service to others eluded me. I thought of nursing as the avenue to a professional career with intrinsic rewards that come with using intellectual skills in the service of others, but in a direct way absent from corporate-style work. In spite of not seeking leadership, it has found me. I find that I now direct my desire and need for intrinsic rewards toward others who are providing that care. In essence, they take care of our patients, and I take care of them. I was exposed to the servant leadership model many years ago, and I would identify that style as the basis for other styles I may employ.

Currently, I ask myself the following questions:

- Is formal leadership where I should be?

- Is formal leadership where I want to be?

- Given what some of the literature suggests about a "masculine" style, is my style of leadership going to work in the long run?

- What other styles are appropriate, and if I learn them, will they become authentic?

- Does being a man in this position necessitate overt skill sets that are historically seen as more masculine?

- Do I need mentors and role models?

- Who should be my mentors and role models?

My introduction into this level of leadership is still unfolding, but I am always reminded of the (not uncommon) complaints I made when working in the hospital: The nurse managers and leaders do not understand what is truly going on, they do not understand the latest in patient care, and so on. Obviously, I try to ensure that staff members know that I am clinically relevant and that this is where I initially got my credibility as a new CNO. Ensuring credibility as a clinician was first on my list of things to do when I began this role. As the role here evolves, I find that it is still being defined. The roles of CNO and COO were split before I arrived, with two of us now performing our respective roles (me and the COO, a non-clinician). During this ongoing process, I have had to learn to protect my sphere and not become involved in things not overtly clinical. I guard this sphere vigilantly. Before this personal experience, I was naive to the need for this level of protection of my sphere of responsibilities.

> **NOTE**
>
> *I am often asked to provide leadership in areas that do not directly affect clinical practice, and I wonder whether that results from an overall need for broad leadership among several people or perhaps because I am male in this role (or maybe this is just the way it is). In my first postgraduate role, I saw that the SVP found herself in meetings where leadership was being sought but the topic or concern had little or nothing to do with the clinical care provided in the organization. I found myself occasionally asking why the SVP of clinical operations needed to be involved in such meetings. The issue raises this question: Is there an overall dearth of leadership in health care organizations to the extent that all members of leadership must be involved in all decision-making, regardless of the issue?*

Answering some of the questions I listed earlier, I do find differences in style as I progress in this role. How much of that is gender difference is difficult to determine and perhaps irrelevant.

What I've Learned

I can now look back on my graduate nursing education and on the exhortations to be a leader and understand that the teaching of relevant leadership skills was sorely lacking. Conflict management skills and styles were not taught. The differences between transformation and transactional styles were not taught. I am innately aware that my style of leadership is transformational (in line, I would argue, with the servant model), which Ayman, Korabik, and Morris (2009) have written tends to be devalued by male subordinates. If this is true, then within nursing the transformational style should be readily welcomed given the gender disparity. But according to Johnson, Murphy, Zewdie, and Reichard (2008), men who exhibit more feminine leadership styles (like transformational styles) tend to be seen as less effective generally. So, the quandary is just that: a man with a more feminine leadership style leading a group of nurses consisting mostly of females. Does it work? The jury is out.

At this point in my formal role, I rely on listening skills and intellect and my natural curiosity to ask questions and keep abreast of current literature in nursing. I now also read books and articles on leadership in general and on clinical leadership in particular. I also now understand that part of my role is threefold: to set a forward-thinking clinical agenda for the organization, by applying evidence-based practice, by considering the direction of future of nursing, and by weighing the current needs of this particular kind of practice. Compared to others at my level in the organization, I do not overtly overreact to events that need attention. Even if such events have immediacy, I maintain a "poker face" even as I am already contemplating solutions.

So, the question of leadership style effectiveness imposes itself daily. If good outcomes are a measure of successful leadership, then whatever style works is quite possibly an answer, but perhaps not the only one. However, with mentoring from others, even better outcomes may be possible. That I ask the question about mentoring indicates that mentoring is welcome, either out of some degree of need for validation or a desire for a colleague with similar professional challenges or, more likely, a combination of both. But as a man in a still predominantly female profession, is gender important in the choice of a mentor? Or should I just evaluate other chief nurses' outcomes and seek them out, regardless of gender?

According to van Engen and Willemsen (2004), transformational leadership style, the style with which I most identify, is more feminine, but it only poses problems if you are out of role (meaning, not female). They write that transactional leadership is a more masculine style. I can only assume that men in nursing leadership are fine as long as we demonstrate typical male characteristics of transactional leadership. However, as Billing and Alversson (2000) have written, we gain little by labeling leadership as feminine or masculine.

NOTE

For example, I find the PDSA (plan, do, study, act) model of quality improvement tedious. Is that because I am male and men are more action-oriented? Or is it just me, regardless of gender? I tend to like quicker iterations of quality initiatives than the PDSA allows. My style is more informal when it comes to quality initiatives: Create a plan, test it, get preliminary data, and tweak it for the next go round.

Ultimately, I question how we are preparing nurse leaders, regardless of gender. Should gender be a part of the equation? I argue probably yes, at least for the time being. Given that nursing is still overwhelmingly female, to ignore some possible gender-specific differences is to ignore the diversity needed in all professions, not just in nursing. Given the overwhelming female presence in nursing, recognition of male and female ways of being could be useful.

Intuitively, I know and welcome official and unofficial mentoring by both genders. I have received excellent words of wisdom from strong female leadership and knew instinctively that it was gender-free advice. At the same time, some level of camaraderie among other men in nursing leadership would have been welcomed. I felt the need for it when I graduated with my undergraduate nursing degree, experienced it again at the graduate level, and experienced it daily when I practiced it at the bedside. I even feel the need for it in my current leadership role.

However, men in nursing and nursing leadership really do have to create it on their own. What I did was to first join the only men in nursing organization I could find—the American Assembly for Men in Nursing (AAMN). Curiously, I had to find it on my own. Mentors in nursing school never identified how that might be an avenue for the minority males in nursing school to find male mentors. Really no other formal avenues to find this kind of professional gender-based camaraderie exist for male nurses.

DO WE REALLY NEED THE AAMN?

The question has been asked before at AAMN whether we actually need a gender-based nursing organization. I conclude there is, but it is obvious our primarily female nursing faculty do not identify the men in the school as having any male-identified mentoring. The need a group like AAMN fulfills is simple. Imagine if you are the only female in a room of professional colleagues, most of whom are practicing in ways that seem "masculine." How does that solitary female react to that experience? Men in nursing are used to being one of the few men in a room at a conference, at a meeting, anywhere. It is at the very least refreshing and energy-filling to be surrounded by mostly men at a meeting and allow for a masculine problem-solving approach to manifest itself.

When I ask myself if, in terms of becoming a leader, coming to nursing later in life was a good thing, I have to answer in the affirmative. I observed leadership styles all along in my earlier non-health care worlds, and I brought those observations with me to nursing. To produce the kind of leadership needed in nursing, current leaders in nursing, even those who stumble into leadership roles as clinicians, need to explore and teach both gender-neutral and gender-identified leadership styles.

MEN IN NURSING SURVIVAL TIPS

If you are coming from another career, be aware of the skills you bring with you.

Find a leadership style that's a comfortable fit for you—regardless of gender assumptions.

Seek professional male camaraderie and mentorship.

Allow your career to go in directions you may not have imagined, despite any gender considerations.

Do not apologize for what are considered more masculine approaches to direct patient care or leadership. Patients and health care organizations are best served when both gender-neutral and gender-identified approaches are brought to bear.

References

Ayman, R., Korabik, K., & Morris, S. (2009). Is transformational leadership always perceived as effective? Male subordinates' devaluation of female transformational leaders. *Journal of Applied Social Psychology, 39*(4), 852-879.

Billing, Y. D., & Alvesson, M. (2000). Questioning the notion of feminine leadership: A critical perspective on the gender labeling of leadership. *Gender, Work and Organization, 7*(3), 144-157.

Grena, P., & Lauve, R. (2006, July/August). Disruptive clinician behavior: A persistent threat to patient safety. *Patient Safety & Quality Healthcare*. Retrieved from http://www.psqh.com/julaug06/disruptive.html

Johnson, S., Murphy, S., Zewdie, S., & Reichard, R. (2008). The strong, sensitive type: Effects of gender stereotypes and leadership prototypes on the evaluation of male and female leaders. *Organizational Behavior and Human Decision Processes, 106*(1), 39-60.

Moran, P., Duffield, C. M., Donoghue, J., Stasa, H., & Blay, N. (2011). Factors impacting on career progression for nurse executives. *Contemporary Nurse, 38*(1-2), 45-55.

Rosenstein, A., & O'Daniel, M. (2008). Survey of the impact of disruptive behaviors and communication defects on patient safety. *Joint Commission Journal on Quality and Pateient Safety, 34*(8), 464–471.

Saxton, R., Hines, T., & Maithe, E. (2009). The negative impact of nurse-physician disruptive bahavior on patient safety: A review of the literature. *Journal of Patient Safety, 5*(3), 180–183.

Tracey, C., & Nicholl, H. (2006). Mentoring and networking: Caroline Tracey and Honor Nicholl consider the value to nursing leadership development of mentoring and networking. *Nursing Management, 12*(10), 28-32.

van Engen, M. L., & Willemsen, T. M. (2004). Sex and leadership styles: A meta-analysis of the research published in the 1990s. *Psychological Reports, 94*(1), 318.

Chapter 3

Leading in a Complex Health Care Environment

Brent MacWilliams, PhD, ANP
Assistant Professor
ACCEL Leadership: Research and Evaluation
University of Wisconsin Oshkosh, College of Nursing

The U.S. health care system is in a profound state of flux as the Patient Protection and Affordable Care Act (PPACA) changes the nature of health care delivery. The landmark Institute of Medicine (IOM) report *The Future of Nursing: Leading Change, Advancing Health* calls for a professional transformation in nursing. Nursing leaders in the academic and clinical settings face a rapidly changing health care system in which nursing professions are charged with "leading change and advancing health" (IOM, 2010). For nursing leaders to meet these new responsibilities, they need to view change through the lens of an equal or full partner in health care delivery (IOM, 2010).

Male nurses interested in becoming leaders are well positioned to meet these new responsibilities as change agents. Men are poorly represented in the nursing workforce but well represented in leadership roles. Male nurses who want to move into leadership roles must embrace a nursing educational and workplace culture that has historically treated men as less-than-full members of the profession. Men have a long history in nursing but a poor track record for retention in nursing school and in the workplace. Men continue to face significant educational barriers and role stress based on latent discrimination and stereotyping. Questions related to the nature of male touch and the ability of men to care in the traditional sense have resulted in the movement of men into "high-tech, low-touch" nursing roles (MacWilliams, Schmidt, & Bleich, 2012). Female educators and coworkers may not sympathize with men being treated as "different" from their peers in the profession when men have traditionally held positions of privilege in almost every other facet of professional life.

Women currently account for nearly half the workforce in the health professions other than nursing (medicine, pharmacy, and physical therapy), and workforce parity for women based on the numbers represents a passing issue (Barzansky & Etzel, 2011). That said, women still face gender-based limitations in the workplace. Images of female nurses being subservient to the physician or typecast as sex objects serve to tarnish the image of the profession and negate value. Likewise, male nurses portrayed as failed caregivers or suspect when providing care that requires intimate touch are symptoms of an oppressed profession. Research shows that men enter nursing for the same reason as women: They hold personal values (like caring for others) that are consistent with the holistic approach in nursing. Men who are nurses and seek leadership roles must be aware of and sensitive to the fact that inequities on social and professional levels still exist for both male and female nurses (MacWilliams et al., 2012).

Nursing leaders must be aware of the issues and help nursing move forward empowered with a gender-blind eye of inclusion. Being a member of a female-dominated profession and facing the social pressure of a nontraditional gender role is stressful, but it also provides men with an intimate understanding of oppression.

The intimate and civilized oppression of men in nursing by women through passive-aggressive behavior leaves *both* parties disempowered (Dong & Temple, 2011):

> *"Persons from oppressed or subordinate groups tend to be more able than those who are in power to perceive and recognize the habits, customs, moods and attitudes and idiosyncrasies of the oppressor. . . . [W]hen persons are denied power and status they will often develop their perceptive abilities as means of coping." (Hanna, Talley, & Guindon, 2000, p. 433)*

Books written to teach men coping/survival techniques in nursing reflect the oppression that still exists (O'Lynn, 2012). Men who practice nursing, despite the adversity they often face, have a unique perspective because they both value the profession and hold the expectation of being a full member of the professional health care team. If nursing is going to assume a leadership role in health care, men are ready to help. If the goal for nursing is professional transformation and becoming full partners in health care, nursing leadership must commit to a fundamental reassessment of professional identity, work out of a diagnosis of oppression, formulate a new care plan of professional empowerment, and commit to measurable outcomes. If nurses do not hold a professional self-respect on par with physicians and other health care professionals, little will change, and patient care will ultimately suffer. Men interested in holding a leadership role in the academic and hospital settings must be aware of past oppression but be ready to move forward with the goal of helping all nurses to work to their full potential (Pope, 2008).

Empowering Nurses to Lead

The IOM's *Future of Nursing* report reads like a care plan for empowerment, imploring nurses to "practice at the full extent of their education and training" (IOM, 2010, p. 85). Nursing leaders must assess the individual needs within their area of responsibilities/expertise, explore strategies to implement needed change and continuously reevaluate the plan, and measure outcomes. Two key messages from the report should direct leadership efforts in academic/hospital settings:

> "**Recommendation 2**: Expand opportunities for nurses to lead and diffuse collaborative improvement efforts. Private and public funders, health care organizations, nursing education programs, and nursing associations should expand opportunities for nurses to lead and manage collaborative efforts with physicians and other members of the health care team to conduct research and to redesign and improve practice environments and health systems. These entities should also provide opportunities for nurses to diffuse successful practices." (IOM, 2010, p. 40)

> "**Recommendation 7**: Prepare and enable nurses to lead change to advance health. Nurses, nursing education programs, and nursing associations should prepare the nursing workforce to assume leadership positions across all levels, while public, private, and governmental health care decision makers should ensure that leadership positions are available to and filled by nurses." (IOM, 2010, p. 43)

The IOM is asking the nursing profession to become a full partner in health care redesign and to take a leadership seat at the health care table. The question is, though, whether nursing is going to sit down. Being more assertive is a social role expectation for men and can bring value to the nursing profession. Power or control is a primary need for human beings, but when power is used without empathy or compassion, it is by definition oppression (Hanna et al., 2000). In most cases, men are the perpetrators of oppressive behavior, but in nursing a culture of female-perpetrated oppression accounts for the mistreatment of both female and male nursing students (eating our young) and lateral workforce violence in which the oppressed become the oppressor (Hanna et al., 2000; Pope, 2008). If the nursing profession fails to break this cycle and fails to embrace a diverse and changing health care landscape, it will fail in its new leadership role.

What Does a Nursing Leadership Profile Look Like?

The traditional command leadership/power model, which emphasizes compliancy and control, is ineffective in today's health care and educational systems. If nursing leaders want to help reshape health care and reform education, they must be empowered, authentic, team-oriented, inclusive, innovative, and competent (American Organization of Nurse Executives [AONE], 2011). Empowerment by any leader is possible only when the leader has the capacity to demonstrate empowering behaviors. Understanding and transcending oppression is a mandate if authenticity and transparency are to be achieved. Transformational leaders have personal power and esteem built on an ethical foundation of keeping those in their charge at the center of the process. Nursing leadership has been asked "to lead and manage collaborative efforts with physicians and other members of the healthcare team to conduct research and to redesign and improve practice environments and health systems" (IOM, 2010, p. 40).

Tapping into Emotional Intelligence

Aspiring nurse leaders must begin this process with a personal journey of exploration and education. Many men who explore nursing as a career hold a measure of emotional intelligence (EI), something often recognized by a career coach (a mother, father sister, brother, aunt, or someone else) who believes that they would make good caregivers. Tapping into the EI skill set keeps the emerging leader grounded in the reality of people as holistic beings and confirms a visceral capacity to engage with people in authentic transactions. Authenticity as a nursing leader requires EI built on a foundation of the following:

- **Self-awareness:** How emotions guide decisions

- **Self-management:** Mastering emotions when adapting to change

- **Social awareness:** The ability to comprehend group dynamics and react to create positive change

- **Relationship management:** Managing change/conflict to create positive adaptation

(Goleman, 1998; Sanford, 2009)

Nursing leaders who have a well-developed and managed EI will have a wonderful life and always have a venue to practice their art.

Self-awareness enables leaders to receive feedback about their strengths and weaknesses without such feedback becoming a personal affront. Instead, leaders see the feedback as an opportunity to improve. A self-aware leader who embraces setbacks along with successes as learning experiences enjoys self-acceptance and confidence. A confident leader allows space for team members to take risk without retribution, which is paramount when change is needed. Transformational leaders are transparent and openly acknowledge that they have made many mistakes. That self-forgiveness provides room for others to make mistakes and improve. Leadership is lost when blame is the outcome measure; improvement through accountability creates fluid and achievable benchmarks. Demonstration of professional nursing values is predicated on self-awareness and the accountability to self-manage that comes with it.

Self-management, an active process, begins with the assessment of your personal and professional goals. A nursing leader's ability to career plan and follow through on those plans is certainly a prerequisite for providing advice and mentoring to peers and subordinates. "Do as I say not as I do" destroys credibility.

Social awareness refers to the ability to comprehend group dynamics and to react to create positive change and draws from the artful side of nursing leaders. For example, the historical dominant/subservient social roles between physicians and nurses often results in conflict. Physicians expect orders to be followed. Nurses often feel powerless and uninvolved in the plan of care, and emotions take over. A nurse with honed EI skills uses emotion to direct the focus away from personal control and shift the focus back towards the care of the patient. The outcome is a more respectful and patient-centered team approach. Cultivation of EI skills provides the toolkit needed for the art of relations management.

Relationship management requires assessment of an emerging leader's strength and weaknesses to provide a baseline to understand the types of positions that best suit his or her skill set and how to identify and empower a team through clearly identified complementary skill sets. Expert coaches are aware that carefully chosen teams with complementary skill sets are often more successful than the "best of the best" who lack a group identity (Rath & Conchie, 2008).

Promoting Inclusion and Collaboration

Emerging nursing leaders who are men understand the need for a more inclusive and collaborative profession. Nursing leaders must commit to removing the barriers for men who want to enter the profession and thus increase the pipeline of all underrepresented student populations. Providing all underrepresented student populations with the tools needed to be a successful member of the health care team must be a metrics-driven mandate. If nursing leaders fail to recognize, value, and embrace differences within the profession, the ability to act in a lead role with the other professions will be lost. Nursing leaders working from a framework of oppression or latent discrimination will be "benched" as they are quickly recognized by staff, physicians, patients, and community stakeholders as disingenuous. The expectation of inclusion must be reflected in metrics that span from admission to completion of nursing school and from the bedside to the boardroom. Knowledge of cultural practice can be appreciated, but competency is a function of the workforce reaching a number that reflects the patient population served. Cultural change is best accomplished when people who differ interact face to face on a regular basis and are immersed in a culture of mutual respect. The nursing profession has made strides toward empowerment and inclusion, but leadership must commit to *benchmark change or get benched*. Men represent 8.9% of the nursing profession yet constitute 49% of the population served (U.S. Bureau of Labor Statistics, 2011). What messages does that send to the other professions? *Do as I say not as I do?*

Innovating

The nursing leader must also be an innovator. Synonymous with change, innovation requires nursing leaders to challenge the status quo and champion projects that range from continuous quality improvement initiatives to models of care that change the nature of health care delivery. The profile of a 21st-century nursing leader is a confident, authentic, team-oriented, collaborative risk taker who is credible through competence (AONE, 2011). The 21st-century nursing leader's dashboard will be filled with nontraditional projects and expectations, but decision making must remain grounded in professional values and behaviors that reflect student/patient-centered care.

What Does the Nursing Leadership Role Require?

Effective communication stands as the cornerstone of relations management. Nursing leaders must be well educated and have the ability to offer oral arguments as well as produce cogent and persuasive written materials. You'll find the ability to communicate effectively key to establishing and maintaining credibility within an interdisciplinary team.

Nurse leaders must also work out of a theoretical framework that creates interdisciplinary synergy. Systems theory serves that purpose well. Nursing's greatest professional strength is providing patient-centered care generated from the holistic nursing perspective. Systems theory, which has evolved into complex adaptive systems (CAS) theory, reflects this holistic perspective, and all nursing leaders should use it for mental modeling. Systems theory is transdisciplinary and provides a common framework of analysis for stakeholders to view the interaction of complex systems such as health care.

Systems-thinking is expansive rather than reductive; it enables leaders to analyze change in a holistic context, which then provides them a better understanding of the downstream effects of any changes made. CAS can help leaders model/simulate change processes and predict effect. For example, the human body is a CAS and adapts systematically to stress in an effort to maintain balance. The hospital is also a CAS, and when staffing changes are made on the medical/surgical floor, those changes place stress on the system. The emergency department (ED) doctors must wait longer to admit patients to the floor; the outcome is that both the ED doctors and patients waiting to be admitted are dissatisfied. Systems theory creates a common framework for interdisciplinary and integrated planning. In systems theory, organizational equilibrium can be assessed. Depending on the practice setting, nursing leaders must be knowledgeable about delivery models and design, health care economics, health care policy, governance, patient safety, case management, risk management, and quality improvement (Clancy, Effken, & Pesut, 2008).

> **NOTE**
>
> *The experienced clinician considering a leadership role in nursing should also consider advanced practice or doctoral education to provide the knowledge base to be a skilled leader. Physicians, pharmacists, and physical therapists all require doctoral preparation as their minimal education, and comparable preparation breeds mutual respect.*

Nursing leaders in both the academic and clinical settings must also master change management. Significant change in any education or practice setting is often met with resistance and conflict. The Lewin change model of unfreezing-change-refreezing is a simple but effective method to guide the process. Unfreezing requires a catalyst as impetus for change. Suppose, for example, that you are the chief executive officer of a large health care system and a climate survey reveals that disruptive behavior by physicians toward nurses is undermining patient care. Organizing a town hall meeting with all parties present to discuss what constitutes disruptive behavior creates a dialogue and accountability through a transparent process. To refreeze the change, review the zero-tolerance policy for disruptive behavior, reinforce the expectation for reporting, and close with a commitment by administration to fair enforcement. Staying on the ethical path as a nursing leader will inevitably create conflict situations, and maintaining control is essential. Emerging nurse leaders must learn to be curious when emotions are running high and consider tactical versus defensive measures to defuse problem situations (Marquis & Huston, 2009).

Nursing educators have done a poor job providing students with conflict management skills. Male students who question nursing instructors are often labeled as troublemakers and treated harshly. Nursing students must be empowered through a more comprehensive value-minded education. Negotiating skills in which conflict is managed in ways that result in positive outcomes will provide students with tools to negotiate conflict within health care settings. Nursing instructors and preceptors often offer covert strategies to maneuver physicians as examples for nursing students; such examples only serve to reinforce a nursing role of subservience and limit the clear expectation for full collaboration between nurses and doctors. Conflict management requires the use of an interest-based approach that focuses on the interests or needs that serve as the basis for the conflict rather than winning the battle. Having students participate in patient care simulations that deal with conflict resolution is an ideal teaching approach.

In addition, nursing leaders must help students to master self-care; otherwise, they will feel inept and lack confidence to work effectively as a change agent. Nurses are charged with teaching self-care, and if they haven't mastered those skills themselves that can translate to a lack of authenticity.

Self-advocacy is a core competency for all nursing students. Providing authentic patient-centered care begins with nursing leaders who empower and advocate for the students and nurses they lead. A nurse who demonstrates self-worth, self-advocacy, and unquestioned patient advocacy within a framework of professional competence and altruism knows the value of nursing practice (Bandura, 1994).

Focusing on Quality

Quality initiatives are the property of nursing; nurses are the masters of outcome measures and maintaining patient satisfaction, which drives change in the PPACA era of health care delivery. The education of nursing leaders should begin with an understanding of the quality initiatives that set nursing apart. Quality and Safety Education of Nurses (QSEN) is a perfect starting point; patient-centered care, teamwork and collaboration, evidence-based practice, quality improvement, safety and informatics are all designed to continuously improve the quality and safety of the health care system (The QSEN Institute). The focus of nursing school on individual patient care in the acute setting as the starting point for nursing students needs to be reframed. Nursing care is shifting to a systems view and community focus, and education must follow.

From a leadership perspective, the number of nursing programs and the quality of those programs also pose a threat to the long-term health of the profession. The profit motivation of proprietary schools calls quality and professional socialization into question. Nursing leaders in academia should focus less on the number of nursing students and consider the quality. Many nursing schools have adopted a holistic admission process that attracts students who hold a capacity as scientists and personal values that align with the values of the nursing profession. Nursing leaders in education must focus on a high-quality nursing education that helps close the theory/practice gap that the workplace demands. Mentorships and clinical residencies help to create a seamless transition for students entering clinical practice, which increases the quality of patient care (IOM, 2010).

In the acute care setting, discussions about labor cost (nursing being the largest) and the quality of patient outcomes have often taken place independently of each other, but that is changing. The baby boomer population (silver tsunami) is arriving to the health care marketplace with the expectation of safe high-quality care. Nursing leaders in the clinical setting must balance safe and high-quality care with delivery cost. Staffing shortages of nurses coupled with unrealistic expectations of higher quality care has given rise to innovation. The Magnet Accreditation Program is the perfect example of quality through empowerment. Nursing leadership representation is expected in the organizational committee structure and executive leadership—coupled with a shared governance management structure. The expectation of collegial working relationships among disciplines creates a flat management profile that breeds equity.

Nurse leaders in academic settings must showcase their research skills; the Interdisciplinary Nursing Quality Research Initiative (INQRI) serves as a perfect example. The INQRI is process oriented, focusing on care coordination, medication administration, and evidence-based protocols that relate directly to nursing care and patient outcomes. Hospital administrators are finding out that they need to "take full advantage of nurses' knowledge and commitment to their patients and institutions—to increase the safety and reliability, patient-centeredness, and efficiency of care" (Needleman & Hassmiller, 2009, p. 633; Sherman & Pross, 2010).

Finding Nursing's Political Empowerment

Historically, the medical profession has enjoyed high social status and self-regard and has been the dominating influence in health care. Physicians have controlled their destiny through a combination of autonomous practice and strong professional organizations like the American Medical Association (AMA). Over the past couple of decades, however, things have changed. For example, membership in the AMA has dropped to 35%, and although the medical profession is highly visible as figureheads in health care, they are only one of many stakeholders, and physician political power might be more of an illusion than a reality (Timmermans & Oh, 2010).

Why is this important? Because many nurses assume that physicians hold the most significant political power in health care, but that is not true. The nursing workforce accounts for the largest percentage of health care providers, with 2.9 million members, and holds a significant political seat based on access, value, and quality care. However, nursing professionals have been apathetic about participating in meaningful political activity and engagement (Sheehan, 2010). Nurses have historically viewed power and the exertion of power as inconsistent with the self-identities as women. Men bring into the profession a chance to redefine the nursing identity as a more diverse and politically active force. The reluctance to embrace empowerment activities may explain the inability to control independent practice (Manojlovich, 2007). Empowered nursing leaders in the academic and clinical setting must fully understand the issues, laws, and health policy critical to increasing independent practice. Nursing students must become politically aware and empowered to manage injustice. Students mentored to view patient advocacy as extending from the bedside to the White House will be more likely to take political action seriously. If nursing leaders fail to take a lead role in political action and the art of exerting influence, nursing will continue to be a pawn in a health care business plan, and patient care will suffer (Sheehan, 2010).

Establishing Value

A Gallup poll has identified nursing again as the *most trusted profession* (Gallup, 2012). But is it one of the most *highly valued* professions? The challenge of nursing leaders is to attach monetary value or savings directly to nursing services to establish measurable value. Nursing has done well establishing value in the case manager arena based on quality outcomes provided by nurses at the bedside. However, nursing aides and unlicensed personnel now perform many of the services traditionally provided by nurses. Successful business-minded nursing leaders abound, but the nursing profession as a whole fails to appreciate health care as a business, one which must justify cost for service. The nursing profession holds the public trust but has not established public value in monetary terms. In the acute care setting, nursing services are often packaged as a room charge, which is a travesty. Health care and education have become billable commodities, and nursing leaders must embrace this as reality. Nursing care outside of the billable care provided by advanced practice nurses (anesthetists, nurse practitioners, and midwives) is minimal at best (Rutherford, 2012).

As a key strategy, nursing leaders need to establish billable value for nursing services based on quality indicators tied directly to nursing practice/service with the goal of establishing independent monetary value.

> **NOTE**
>
> *The PPACA is funding grants to support the delivery of evidence-based and community-based prevention and wellness services This would be a perfect opportunity for nursing to study and establish billable value through evidence-based prevention activities that reduce chronic disease, especially in underserved areas (Kaiser Family Foundation, 2010).*

If nursing does not establish value for specific services/plans of care, the practice of nurses providing direct patient care will continue to erode. Nursing leaders in the academic setting with research skills need to partner with health care agencies to investigate all facets of providing quality patient care. Interdisciplinary studies that relate directly to increasing patient safety are a priority (like the reduction of medication errors). Research results that show a quantifiable increase in patient safety that are directly attributable to nursing practice establish value. The results of Laurant et al.'s (2009) systematic review revealed similar outcomes and potential cost savings with appropriately trained advanced practice nurses, compared to primary care physicians, which serves to establish value. Nurse practitioners are embracing their new leadership role, and patients wanting to access primary care are finding nurse practitioners at the door. In the new Medicare Medical Home Demonstration Project, nursing practitioners serve as the case managers and care providers who offer patients access and integrated care planning (Schram, 2010).

Nursing leaders in the academic setting spend too little time discussing the business side of health care even with students enrolled in graduate programs who will have direct fiscal responsibilities. Nursing students need to become aware early in the educational process that caring costs money, that the services they provide are valuable, and that documentation of services is a professional responsibility. Health care over the past half century has been transformed into a pay-for-disease-service marketplace driven by reimbursement for medical services. PPACA has changed the game, and the door is open for nursing to place monetary value on holistic and prevention-based outcomes. The baby boomers are accessing health care in large numbers and expect to be treated as a consumer and have positive outcomes; nursing can deliver on both.

Nursing over the past half century has remained committed to altruism and to act in the best interest of the patient while business-focused professionals scrambled for market share. The reality is that nursing services do come at a cost that must be quantified. Men who are nurses and want to establish themselves as leaders in the 21st-century health care system must be business-minded without losing track of the professional values and behaviors that have established nursing as the most trusted profession. Nursing leaders must clarify the value of nursing services while maintaining a moral compass with patient/student-centered care as magnetic north.

Nurses Leading into the Future

The IOM's *Future of Nursing* report clearly identifies nursing as the profession best equipped to lead health care based on access and value. Health care is a finite and expensive commodity, and with the PPACA offering more people access to services, nursing is positioned to provide cost-effective, outcome-based services. Forward-thinking nursing leaders in both the academic and clinical setting should see opportunities daily to improve service delivery.

Authentic nursing leaders are confident, authentic, assertive, team oriented, collaborative, risk takers, and credible through competence. Leaders' decision making must also be grounded in professional values and behaviors that reflect student/patient-centered care. Nursing leaders in academic setting must produce research that has practice applicability or that empowers nursing students to self-advocate, embrace change, and provide safe high-quality care (AONE, 2011).

The health care system of the past was based on a business model that thrived on billing for procedures with limited accountability for outcomes, but things have changed. The PPACA has new accountabilities related to readmissions. Services provided in the acute care setting are becoming quality focused and cost-effective, which is shifting care back to the community setting. Acute care facilities are moving to home-health models that focus on prevention and high-quality care to limit the length of stay and number of hospital readmissions. Nursing has never left the community, and now health care is coming back to where people live. Nursing leaders must be ready to lead the change. Nursing leadership in academia must adapt their curriculum to account for a different set of expectations as students enter the workforce.

Men who are nurses and interested in leading in this complex health care environment face a unique set of challenges. Men are significantly underrepresented in the nursing profession. The nursing culture has historically not been kind to men, but women have had their own struggles dealing with a professional role that has been subservient to physicians. Nursing is a female-dominated profession, and with the history of women's exclusion from leadership positions, the reaction to more men in nursing leadership roles will be mixed. Men who have stayed in the profession despite the pressures are in a unique position as leaders to help transform the profession and can help nursing take a full partnership seat at the health care table. The message of inclusion is powerful and speaks to a new vision of professional unity, awareness, and accountability through access, value, and quality outcomes. If nursing leaders are going to help transform health care in the 21st century, there must be a new professional maturity that serves to step away from a history of subservience to medicine and assume a new professional identity as a full partner in health care leadership. The IOM report is a care plan of empowerment, and nursing leaders in the academic and clinical setting should use it as a roadmap to navigate the ever-changing health care system. It is the job of nursing leaders to move that work forward in both the educational and workplace settings through a framework of empowerment (Manojlovich, 2007; Porter-O'Grady, 2011).

MEN IN NURSING LEADERSHIP SURVIVAL TIPS

Take advantage of the opportunities in nursing; male nurses are expected to move into leadership roles.

Be inclusive by supporting and empowering your female peers.

Support "zero tolerance" for oppressive behaviors in nursing school and the workplace.

Be politically active and support nursing taking a seat at the health care table.

Become a lifelong learner and use that knowledge to establish nursing as a valued 21st-century profession.

References

American Organization of Nurse Executives (AONE). (2011). *The AONE nurse executive competencies*. Retrieved from http://www.aone.org/resources/leadership%20tools/PDFs/AONE_NEC.pdf

Bandura, A. (1994). Self-efficacy. In V.S. Ramachandran (Ed.), *Encyclopedia of human behavior, 4,* (71-81). New York: Academic Press.

Barzansky, B., & Etzel, S. I. (2011, September 17). Medical schools in the United States, 2010-2011. *JAMA, 306*(9), 1007-1014.

Clancy, T, R., Effken, J., & Pesut, D. (2008). Applications of complex systems theory in nursing education, research and practice. *Nursing Outlook, 56*(5), 248-256, doi: 10.1016/j.outlook.2008.06.010.

Dong, D., & Temple, B. (2011, July-September). Oppression: A concept analysis and implications for nurses and nursing. *Nursing Forum, 46*(3), 169-176. http://dx.doi.org/doi:10.1111/j.1744-6198.2011.00228.x

Gallup. (2012). Honesty/Ethics in Professions [Poll].Retrieved from http://www.gallup.com/poll/1654/honesty-ethics-professions.aspx#1

Goleman, D. (1998). *Working with Emotional Intelligence*. New York: Bantam.

Hanna, F. J., Talley, W. B., & Guindon, M. H. (2000). The power of perception: Toward a model of cultural oppression and liberation. *Journal of Counseling & Development, 78,* 430-441. Retrieved from http://www.dhss.delaware.gov/dsamh/files/perception1192.pdf

Institute of Medicine (IOM). (2010). *The future of nursing: Leading change, advancing health*. Washington, DC: The National Academies Press.

Kaiser Family Foundation. (2010). *Summary of new health reform law; Patient protection and affordable care act (P.L. 111-148)*. Retrieved from http://www.kff.org/healthreform/upload/finalhcr.pdf

Laurant, M., Reeves, D., Hermens, R., Braspenning, J., Grol, R., & Sibbald, B. (2009). Substitution of doctors by nurses in primary care. *Cochrane Database of Systematic Reviews.* http://dx.doi.org/doi: 10.1002/14651858.CD001271.pub2

MacWilliams, B. R., Schmidt, B., & Bleich, M. R. (2013). Men in nursing. *American Journal of Nursing, 113*(1), 38-44. http://dx.doi.org/doi:10.1097/01.NAJ.0000425744.76107.9f

Manojlovich, M. (2007, January). Power and empowerment in nursing: Looking backward to inform the future. *OJIN: The Online Journal of Issues in Nursing,* 12. Retrieved from http://www.nursingworld.org/MainMenuCategories/ANAMarketplace/ANAPeriodicals/OJIN/TableofContents/Volume122007/No1Jan07/LookingBackwardtoInformtheFuture.html?css=print

Marquis, B. L., & Huston, C. J. (2009). *Leadership roles and management functions in nursing: theory and application* (6th ed.). Philadelphia: Wolters Kluwer Health/Lippincott Williams & Wilkins.

Needleman, J., & Hassmiller, S. (2009, June 12). The role of nurses improving hospital quality and efficiency: Real-world results. *Health Affairs, 28*(4), w625-w633. http://dx.doi.org/DOI 10.1377/hlthaff.28.4.w625

O'Lynn, C. (2012). *A man's guide to a nursing career.* New York: Springer Publishing Company.

Pope, B. G. (2008). *Transforming oppression in nursing education: Towards liberation pedagogy* (Doctoral dissertation, University of North Carolina). Retrieved from http://libres.uncg.edu/ir/uncg/listing.aspx?id=356

Porter-O'Grady, T. (2011, May). Leadership at all levels. *Nursing Management, 42*(5), 32-37. http://dx.doi.org/DOI-10.1097/01.NUMA.0000396347.49552.86

The QSEN Institute. (n.d.). Retrieved from http://qsen.org/about-qsen/pilot-schools-june-2007-november-2008/

Rath, T., & Conchie, B. (2008). *Strengths based leadership: Great leaders, teams, and why people follow.* New York: Gallup Press.

Rutherford, M. M. (2012, July-August). Nursing is the room rate. *Nursing Economics, 30*(4), 193-206. Retrieved from https://www.nursingeconomics.net/ce/2014/article3004193206.pdf

Sanford, K. (2009). Overview of nursing leadership. Retrieved from http://scholar.googleusercontent.com/scholar?q=cache:NVLo-C6SRMAJ:scholar.google.com/&hl=en&as_sdt=0,50

Schram, A. P. (2010, February). Medical home and the nurse practitioner: A policy analysis. *The Journal for Nurse Practitioners, 6*(2), 132-139. Retrieved from http://www.canppasadena.org/wp-content/uploads/2009/08/Medical-Homes-Article.pdf

Sheehan, A. (2010). The value of health care advocacy for nurse practitioners. *Journal of Pediatric Health Care, 24*(4), 280-282. http://dx.doi.org/doi:10.1016/j.pedhc.2010.04.001

Sherman, R., & Pross, E. (2010, January 31). Growing future nurse leaders to build and sustain healthy work environments at the unit level. *OJIN: The Online Journal of Issues in Nursing, 15*. Retrieved from http://www.nursingworld.org/MainMenuCategories/ANAMarketplace/ANAPeriodicals/OJIN/TableofContents/Vol152010/No1Jan2010/Growing-Nurse-Leaders.html

Timmermans, S., & Oh, H. (2010, October 8). The continued social transformation of the medical profession. *Journal of Health and Social Behavior, 51*(1), 94-106. http://dx.doi.org/doi:10.1177/0022146510383500

U.S. Bureau of Labor Statistics. (2011). Employed persons by detailed occupation, sex, race, Hispanic or Latino ethnicity [Statistics]. Retrieved from http://www.bls.gov/cps/cpsaat11.pdf

Chapter 4

Men in Nursing: Historical Career Perspectives

Steven A. Marks, MS, RN
Jeffrey L. Bevan, MSN, RN, FNP-BC, CEN

Even though more men are choosing nursing as a profession, many areas of nursing still remain difficult for males to enter. Historically, nursing has been a female-dominated field. According to the U.S. Bureau of Labor Statistics (2010), men represent 8.9% of the U.S. nursing workforce (see Figure 4.1). However, men currently account for 11.4% of students in baccalaureate programs, 9.9% of students in graduate programs, 6.8% of students in research doctorate programs, and 9.4% of practice doctorate programs (American Association of Colleges of Nursing [AACN], 2012). See Figure 4.2. So, progress has been made recently with regard to men making inroads into the nursing demographic, but barriers and stigmas still exist, both in the nursing profession itself and in U.S. society. As this chapter discusses, embracing men in nursing through a culture of inclusion has had mixed results. This chapter explores the following:

- Factors that influence career choice among men in nursing
- Common nontraditional roles for men in nursing

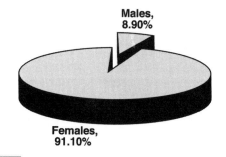

FIGURE 4.1

Percent of male and female nurses in the United States (statistics from U.S. Bureau of Labor Statistics, 2010).

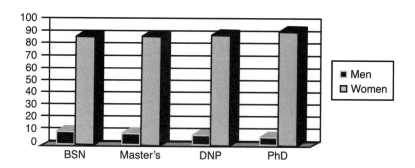

FIGURE 4.2

Percent of male and female students enrolled in nursing programs in the United States (statistics from American Association of Colleges of Nursing, 2012).

As a male in the nursing profession, successful navigation of competing career choices depends on your careful understanding of the culture and norms within each nursing specialty. Although some career barriers still exist, you will find many benefits to being a male nurse.

Why Do Men Enter the Nursing Profession?

Compared with other career choices available to men, nursing can provide job security, a good salary, career mobility, and career advancement (Rambur, Palumbo, McIntosh, Cohen, & Naud, 2011; Tracey & Nicholl, 2007).

- Considering the recent levels of global economic instability, choosing a career that has flexible hours and that cannot be outsourced to a foreign country is a smart move.

- Another trend that might encourage you as a man to choose nursing is how receptive nursing is to those choosing it as a second career. Those who bring skills from other disciplines, such as business, finance, or IT, will find that those skills interface particularly well with nursing careers; they can help you navigate a rapidly changing and expanding health care environment.

- Finally, the aging of America coupled with a relative projected shortage of professional nurses makes nursing a profession well-positioned to accommodate career-oriented men who want to assume roles at bachelor's, master's, and doctoral levels.

> ### SECOND-CAREER NURSES: MAKING YOUR FIRST CAREER SKILLS WORK FOR YOUR
>
> *Nurses coming from a business background will find their budgeting, leadership, employee relations, and customer service skills apply to nursing department operations.*
>
> *Nurses with IT experience will find their programming or tech support skills can be used in nursing informatics to help improve documentation efficiencies.*
>
> *Nurses who bring strong financial backgrounds, like from a financial analyst or CPA background, could use their skills in accounting, cost-containment, or purchasing capacities.*

The most influential factors for deciding to become a nurse include advice from practicing nurses, parental support, and support of friends or peers (Buerhaus, Donelan, Norman, & Dittus, 2005; Goddard, 1999). As expected, male nurses' first exposure to the nursing profession occurs in prelicensure nursing school. Unfortunately, some men do not find the experience enjoyable, nor do these students find many male role models (Ellis, Meeker, & Hyde, 2006; Ierardi, Fitzgerald, & Holland, 2010). Further, male students had experiences of standing out more in class; being stereotyped as gay, effeminate, or less caring; being seen as important for patient lifting (muscle); and often being asked when they were planning to attend medical school (Bartfay, Bartfay, Clow, & Wu, 2010; Hart, 2005; Meadus & Twomey, 2011). Based on these reported experiences, we see opportunities to improve male nurses' entrance into the profession by:

1. Designing educational environments that are supportive of male student nurses' learning needs

2. Providing mentoring opportunities with male nursing faculty both during prelicensure education and after as the student transitions into practice

Nursing appeals to a broad range of ages and needs. If you are a younger male entering the nursing profession, the job's career mobility may be of greater importance to you than other factors. If you are an older male, you might desire stability and a good salary that nursing can provide. However, one could argue that younger men in a female-dominated field face a greater challenge because of the social expectation of men doing "men's work." As more men enter nursing, this issue might attenuate over time. An experienced male intensive care unit (ICU) nurse recently recalled that earlier in his career patients would comment about their uncertainty of having a male nurse provide their care. Over time, however, patients reported that they enjoyed male nurses providing their care, some even preferring men over women for their nursing care.

As the United States and many other countries struggle with the economic downturn, health care is one area that may lend itself to better career and financial stability. Males often enter the nursing profession as a second career or after a midlife career change. With the median wage for registered nurses (RNs) at $65,950 (U.S. Bureau of Labor Statistics, 2011) and the opportunity to make more than $100,000 in advanced practice and administrative roles, a nursing career can provide life-long opportunity. From working as a bedside care nurse (where the vast majority of nurses start their career) to teaching or doing research, men can find fields within nursing that vary with their career desires.

CAREER SPOTLIGHTS

Steve F., MSN, RN

Building on a successful career as a staff nurse and house supervisor for the past 15 years, Steve has channeled his passion for information technology in hopes of bringing a multidisciplinary perspective to health care information

continues

systems to improve nursing care and patient safety. In addition to his BSN, Steve completed a bachelor's degree in information technology and has an MSN with a focus on nursing informatics. As an informatician, Steve plans to utilize his diverse background in nursing to bring real-world experience to developing nurse-friendly electronic health records. Steve comments, "Often, electronic health records are developed around the technology used to create them. I want to see transformation in the industry, where the user experience is seamless and intuitive."

Matt H., RN

Matt, a nurse for nearly 20 years, found success as an emergency department nurse and as a nursing supervisor in acute care hospitals. The lessons learned during those years prepared Matt well for the role he has today. He currently serves as a Program Director for a multistate aeromedical service. Matt credits his success to building relationships with many people throughout his nursing career, as well as the foundational skills he learned in nursing school, such as effective communication and the necessity of effective teamwork for the delivery of products and services. He also relates that his career success is defined by much more than his nursing knowledge: "You do not need to know everything to be 'the best' in nursing; a great attitude and personality are much more important."

Where Do Men Typically Start Their Nursing Career?

Men usually seek out jobs in the critical-care environments, such as ICUs, emergency departments, and perioperative settings. Currently, a dearth of data supports this assertion, although some evidence suggest that preference for specialty nursing begins in male students' undergraduate nursing programs (Lo & Brown, 2000). Further, no specific data evaluates where men start their nursing careers, a finding that in itself is a cause for concern. However, anecdotal evidence suggests that men tend to seek exciting and intellectually challenging environments. For example, the American Assembly for Men in Nursing (AAMN) 2012 membership survey ($n = 149$) revealed that respondents were primarily holding administrative, clinical, or faculty roles. Most likely areas of study reported by this survey were acute care, adult care, and trauma.

Men may also choose a practice area based on work-life requirements. For example, some jobs support part-time work, 12-hour shifts, shift work, and flexible shift scheduling. The flexibility may be more important than the actual practice area.

As a new nurse, you might have to choose an area that you do not find particularly interesting, but it can serve as an important opportunity to springboard into the position of your choice. For example, you might want to consider working in a medical/surgical unit to get general clinical experience before transferring into other clinical environments that require specialized skills.

Finally, you might find that a nurse manager wants to hire you based on your gender. You'll hear various explanations for this decision, but the bottom line in this: Some of the best teams in health care are, arguably, those where men and women work together. Bygren (2010) found that both men and women employees' probability of leaving a workplace in a variety of disciplines *decreased* with the presence of employees of the opposite gender. In health care environments where both male and female patients seek care, gender diversity in the nursing workforce is important to meet the needs and comfort levels for all patients who present for care. Recently, a male nursing faculty member commented about his experience getting hired as an adjunct faculty member: "When I was hired to work as adjunct faculty, I was asked if I would mind teaching in the LPN program, because there were no male faculty and the dean wanted a male role model for the male students. Of course, I was happy to accept." This is a clear example of how creating gender diverse teams in nursing provides a benefit—in this case, with male nursing students.

Whether in nursing school or as recent graduates, men seek out different areas of nursing based on their clinical interests and work-life needs. Although one might say that people choose any career based on interests and work-life balance, the nursing profession affords some of the greatest career diversity compared to nearly any other professional discipline.

Nontraditional Roles for Men in Nursing

As part of a group that represents about 8.9% of the nursing workforce in the United States (U.S. Bureau of Labor Statistics, 2010), as a male in nursing, you have a lot of great opportunity, and you also face certain limitations at the same time. What does this mean? As a male, you will progress through nursing in certain roles with relative ease; others will prove more difficult. With the myriad ongoing initiatives focused on encouraging men to go into nursing, you would think we could work in any area we want to. However, societal norms, stigma, and the sheer unequal balance of male nurses to female nurses might make it harder for you to get into certain areas of nursing.

Males are underrepresented in a number of areas in nursing. For example, obstetrics (OB) is one area where males nurses seem underrepresented or even absent. For males, OB nursing represents one of the greatest challenges to break into as a career. One probably does not need to speculate too long as to the reasons why—societal norms and patient preferences. Aside from male physicians, you don't see many men working in a labor and delivery (L&D) unit. Are female nurses very protective of this practice area and unwilling to see males as capable OB nurses? Do pregnant women stigmatize men as uncaring, and do they assume a male nurse cannot relate to what they are going through?

The recent past might provide perspective. After all, not that long ago, hospital staff used to kick husbands out of the L&D room during a delivery. Even so, in a study by McRae (2003), 67.6% of pregnant women gave positive responses about a male serving as the primary nurse during labor. Further, 73% of the Association of Women's Health, Obstetric, and Neonatal Nursing (AWHONN) nurse respondents reported positive attitudes regarding men in obstetrics. As more men enter nursing, opportunities will, we hope, increase for men who want to pursue work in these nontraditional roles.

Careful planning is important to seize opportunities as they come your way. According to the AAMN survey cited earlier in this chapter, fewer men work in the following nontraditional roles: women's health, clinical research, family care, oncology, and mental health. Men tend to prefer gender-neutral specialties over those rated highly feminine, such as midwifery, pediatrics, school nursing, medical/surgical, palliative, and oncology (Muldoon & Reilly, 2003).

Why have some areas in nursing become nontraditional for men? The several plausible reasons include the following:

1. Career interest in specialty areas

2. Role strain, as a result of directing men into nursing career paths that are not well-matched with their interests/abilities or that are overly feminine in nature (Brown, 2009)

3. Male nurse preferences to work in environments with other men for socialization reasons (Evans & Frank, 2003)

4. The perception of the role being nonmasculine (Allison, Beggan, & Clements, 2004). This strain occurs when behavior and expectations of male nurses are judged with the social norms and expectations of female nurses within our discipline.

As you consider a nontraditional career path in nursing, be aware that you might encounter gender-specific discrimination. Despite this, though, you should enter a nursing area to which you truly feel drawn! When making your decision, consider your fit as a nursing colleague and other important issues such as the compensation package, work hours, work environment, opportunities for mentoring, and a supportive leadership team.

What Does This Mean for You?

Some evidence suggests that being a male in the nursing profession offers advantages as a minority, including professional power, promotion opportunities (Kleinman, 2004), a higher salary on average than female nurses (Williams, 1995), and primary author credit when publishing studies (Shields, Hall, & Mamun, 2011). Further, Evans (1997) asserts that men are disproportionately represented in administrative positions and specialty positions (for example, emergency, nurse anesthesia) and that men perhaps accomplish this by distancing themselves from female colleagues and the feminine image of the nursing profession.

Whether men's career trajectory in nursing is influenced by societal expectations that men are employed across their adult years and remain in the workforce for longer uninterrupted periods or whether it is a function of responding to barriers brought about through the sexualization of nursing practice as women's work (Evans, 2004; Villeneuve, 1994), it remains clear that men's success is moderated by barriers within and outside of the nursing profession. Future research about male nurse roles as they evolve is warranted.

Recruiting and retaining more men in nursing is essential to meet the needs of today's and tomorrow's diverse and complex patients (Xu, 2008). Priority areas include the following:

1. Incorporating recruitment strategies that focus on men

2. Designing gender-neutral educational experiences and textbooks to teach nursing practice across the life span

3. Utilizing evidence-based mentoring/socialization programs for male nurses

4. Encouraging gender diversity in the workplace

5. Designing interventions that change the public perception of men in nursing (Roth & Coleman, 2008)

Men are well positioned to meet the health needs of a variety of patient populations in diverse practice settings and should focus on important health issues, such as leading men's health initiatives.

IMPORTANT ISSUES FACING MEN:

- *Prostate cancer*
- *Testicular cancer*
- *Obesity, stress, and nutrition*
- *Cardiac-related problems*

MEN IN NURSING SURVIVAL TIPS

You will be stereotyped, but remember you are a qualified nurse regardless of your gender.

Don't let your gender keep you from pursuing the specialization you want.

Advance your education so you stay competitive to advance your career

You can't wait for things to happen to you; you need to make them happen.

Improvise, adapt, and overcome; be flexible and take risks!

References

Allison, S. T., Beggan, J. L., & Clements, C. (2004). Derogatory stereotypic beliefs and evaluations of male nurses. *Equal Opportunities International, 23,* 162-178.

American Association of Colleges of Nursing (AACN). (2012). *New AACN data show an enrollment surge in baccalaureate and graduate programs amid calls for more highly educated nurses.* Retrieved from http://www.aacn.nche.edu/news/articles/2012/enrollment-data

Bartfay, W. J., Bartfay, E., Clow, K. A., & Wu, T. (2010). Attitudes and perceptions towards men in nursing education. *Internet Journal of Allied Health Sciences and Practice, 8*(2), 1-6.

Brown, B. (2009). Men in nursing: Re-evaluating masculinities, re-evaluating gender. *Contemporary Nurse, 33*(2), 120-129.

Buerhaus, P. I., Donelan, K., Norman, L., & Dittus, R. (2005). Nursing students' perceptions of a career in nursing and impact of a national campaign designed to attract people into the nursing profession. *Journal of Professional Nursing, 21*(2), 75-83.

Bygren, M. (2010). The gender composition of workplaces and men's and women's turnover. *European Sociological Review, 26*(2), 193-202.

Ellis, D. M., Meeker, B. J., & Hyde, B. L. (2006). Exploring men's perceived educational experiences in a baccalaureate program. *Journal of Nursing Education, 45*(12), 523-527.

Evans, J. (1997). Men in nursing: Issues of gender segregation and hidden advantage. *Journal of Advanced Nursing, 26*(2), 226-231.

Evans, J. (2004). Men nurses: A historical and feminist perspective. *Journal of Advanced Nursing, 47*(3), 321-328.

Evans, J., & Frank, B. (2003). Contraindications and tensions: Exploring relations of masculinities in the numerically female-dominated nursing profession. *Journal of Men's Studies, 11*(3), 277-292.

Goddard, D. K. (1999). *Occupational stereotyping and its influence on men in nursing.* (Doctoral dissertation). Southern Illinois University, Carbondale, IL.

Hart, K. A. (2005). What do men in nursing really think? *Nursing, 35*(11), 46-48.

Ierardi, J. A., Fitzgerald, D. A., & Holland, D. T. (2010). Exploring male students' educational experiences in an associate degree nursing program. *Journal of Nursing Education, 49*(4), 215-218.

Kleinman, C. S. (2004). Understanding and capitalizing on men's advantages in nursing. *Journal of Nursing Administration, 34*(2), 78-82.

Lo, R., & Brown, R. (2000). Perceptions of nursing students on men entering nursing as a career. *Australian Journal of Advanced Nursing, 17*(2), 36-41.

McRae, M. J. (2003). Men in obstetrical nursing: Perceptions of the role. *Maternal Child Nursing, 28*(3), 167-173.

Meadus, R. J., & Twomey, J. C. (2011). Men student nurses: The nursing education experience. *Nursing Forum, 46*(4), 269-279.

Muldoon, O. T., & Reilly, J. (2003). Career choice in nursing students: Gendered constructs as psychological barriers. *Journal of Advanced Nursing, 43*(1), 93-100.

Rambur, B., Palumbo, M. V., McIntosh, B., Cohen, J., & Naud, S. (2011). EXTRA: Young adults' perception of an ideal career: Does gender matter? *Nursing Management, 42*(4), 19-24.

Roth, J. E., & Coleman, C. L. (2008). Perceived and real barriers for men entering nursing: Implications for gender diversity. *Journal of Cultural Diversity, 15*(3), 148-152.

Shields, L., Hall, J., & Mamun, A. A. (2011). The 'gender gap' in authorship in nursing literature. *Journal of the Royal Society of Medicine, 104*(11), 457-464.

Tracey, C., & Nicholl, H. (2007). The multifaceted influence of gender in career progress in nursing. *Journal of Nursing Management, 15*(7), 677-682.

U.S. Bureau of Labor Statistics. (2010). Employed persons by detailed occupation, sex, race, and Hispanic or Latino ethnicity, 2010 annual averages (Table 11). Retrieved from http://www. bls.gov/cps/cps_aa2010.htm

U.S. Bureau of Labor Statistics. (2011). Occupational employment and wages, May 2011, registered nurses. Retrieved from http:// www.bls.gov/oes/current/oes291111.htm

Villeneuve, M. J. (1994). Recruiting and retaining men in nursing: A review of the literature. *Journal of Professional Nursing, 10*(4), 217-228.

Williams, C. L. (1995). Hidden advantages for men in nursing. *Nursing Administration Quarterly, 19*(2), 63-70.

Xu, Y. (2008). Men in nursing: Origin, career path, and benefits to nursing as a profession. *Home Health Care Management and Practice, 21*(1), 72-73.

Chapter 5

Men and Mentorship: A Significant Component of Professional Development

Franklin Shaffer, EdD, RN, FAAN
CEO, CGFNS International

The Institute of Medicine's (IOM) highly influential report, *The Future of Nursing: Leading Change, Advancing Health*, noted that among those goals essential to the future of nursing (and not incidentally, the future of health in the United States) is "to improve the quality of patient care, a greater emphasis must be placed on making the nursing workforce more diverse, particularly in the areas of gender and race/diversity" (IOM, 2010, p. 209). Moreover, the report noted that:

> " . . . throughout much of the 20th century, the nursing profession was composed mainly of women. While the absolute number of men who become nurses has grown dramatically in the last two decades, . . . [e]fforts to recruit more men into the civilian nurs-

ing profession have had minimal success . . . .[T]he profession needs to continue efforts to recruit men; their unique perspectives and skills are important to the profession and will help contribute additional diversity to the workforce." (IOM, 2010, p. 127)

Various sociological barriers have traditionally inhibited men from joining nursing as a professional career, thus resulting in a relative absence of male role models in the profession for young men. So, a very real need exists to encourage men who are already nurses to actively mentor young men who are considering the profession, male nursing students, and new graduates. Mentoring has long been recognized as a vital activity, making a critically important contribution to strengthening leadership skills and improving the career of the mentor as well as the career trajectory of mentees. Even just a kind, thoughtful, and intentionally supportive gesture from someone can make a difference in how a person feels about himself and his choice of career.

Mentoring is always a two-way process: a mutually beneficial and interactive partnership. Both participants benefit from the investment of time. This investment often leads to faster career development for both parties, better psychosocial adjustment to the profession or discipline for the mentee, and a rich exchange of ideas for the mentor. One of the key components of a successful, mutually beneficial mentoring relationship is that each participant shares the same or similar values and vision of the profession. As men in nursing, we have a unique position to serve as mentors to other men in nursing, whether they are just starting their career or they have been practicing for years and are now transitioning to another role. We know what it is like to be a male and a nurse and the distinctive challenges that role will undoubtedly entail.

Moreover, successful mentoring leads to increased professional commitment and satisfaction that extends well beyond the mentoring relationship.

> ### AN ENDURING MENTORING RELATIONSHIP
>
> *When I was a graduate student attempting to matriculate to Teacher's College Columbia University, I met an extraordinary teacher, Robert Piemonte. I was fortunate to succeed in having my first course with him as the professor. It was on nursing administration, and what an impact he made on me. It was his last class for the day (late evening), and it seemed as if the most interesting aspects of the content happened towards the end of the session. Invariably I would ask a question at the end that required the class hour to run over. To this day when I see him he reminds me and others of this. I couldn't wait for the week to roll around to attend his class. In the late 70s it was, and even today it still is, rare to find a doctoral-prepared male nurse professor specializing in nursing administration. He has been my mentor and role model ever since that time. I treasure one piece of advice he gave me, and I have passed it along to every one of my mentees: "Everywhere that I have worked, there has always been an opportunity for me to learn more, to increase my value to others and to the organization. If you take advantage of these, you will better yourself." We have remained friends to this day—and he still gives me advice! I am so grateful for Bob.*

Characteristics of Mentors (and Mentees)

Ideally, a mentor reminds us of who we *could be*, of what we are *actually* here for, and how much we *could choose* to contribute. Each person has an instinctive way of experiencing life. Mentors pull us out into a counter-instinctive way of living it, a place where we would not go unless we were dragged there; they pull us into a world of new possibilities. We all like our comfort zones, but the mentor makes us *un*comfortable, stretching us toward something more. The mentee, for his part, has to invest something of himself to get something more in return.

Clearly then, a mentor has to be insightful and both generous and secure in himself, willing to open himself to the possibility of developing *someone else,* of investing his own talents and abilities in the success of *someone else.* The mentor must redefine his role from one of achieving success to one of making a *contribution.* When you redefine your role from personal success to contribution, "it is never a single individual who is transformed. Transformation overrides the divisions of identity and possession …recasting the tight pattern of scarcity into a widespread array of abundance" (Zander & Zander, 2000, p. 61).

DEVELOPING PEOPLE SKILLS—A MENTORING SUCCESS STORY

One young male nursing student whom I mentored was serious and very focused, so much so that he eagerly tried new things or took advantage of new opportunities without even thanking the people who had helped him. To say the least, he was task-oriented rather than people-oriented. He rarely gave a compliment to anyone and smiled even more rarely. He was increasingly distancing others from him to the point they would go out of their way to avoid him. So, in one of my sessions with him, I gave him a set of tasks:

- *To write a thank you note each week to someone who had helped him. In the age of text messages, emails, and Facebook, a handwritten note has even more impact.*

> - *To say something complimentary to at least one colleague every day.*
>
> - *To make a concerted effort to smile when appropriate three times a day.*
>
> *Soon these "tasks" became second nature to him—others noticed the change and his reputation and his opportunities began to soar.*

To benefit from the experience, the mentee has to *trust* the mentor: allowing himself to be pushed out of his comfort zone, having his own instincts challenged, and willingly opening his perspectives to new horizons. So, the ideal mentee can control his competitive instincts, is humble enough to recognize the talents and successes of others, and is secure enough to consider and learn from the suggestions and even criticisms of another. He must willingly reinvent himself and give up measuring himself against the performance of others and instead focus on developing his own inner abilities. Therefore, the mentee must redefine his role from one of achieving success to one of seeking professional fulfillment, with all the enthusiasm and passion that involves. Not everyone can devote himself to the role of mentor, and not everyone wants mentoring.

FROM MENTOR/MENTEE TO FRIENDS AND COLLEAGUES

When I was the Deputy Director of the National League for Nursing (NLN), I was frequently asked to give speeches. At this particular speech, however, I noticed a young man in the audience who was quite literally hanging on every word I said: a not-so-frequent experience!

continues

After the talk, he waited until everyone else had left and then he approached me. He said that he appreciated my presentation, and he asked if there was any way he could intern with me. While NLN did offer some internships, I had another idea. I was creating a new position: an assistant for special projects. He was interested. He applied for the job, and I did hire him. He was so thirsty for knowledge and experience that he was like a sponge. I taught him the difference between association staff and elected officers. I walked him through the politics of nursing organizations. We worked together and wrote together. We have very similar visions and approaches, so much so that he could take my place in meetings and even give speeches for me. I encouraged him to go on to earn his PhD, and he did. Today, he is working in the global arena as a global health care strategist for a multinational corporation. We are still colleagues and friends and I find myself today calling upon him for some advice in the global arena. It is as if we have always known and respected each other.

Social Mentoring on the Web

Mentoring comes in many different flavors: "from formal to informal, group, situational and flash—there is a new type of mentoring exchange that we might call 'social mentorship' which leverages social networks and social media to forge connections among individuals in need of advice, admonition or assistance" (Krzmarzick, 2012). In 2011, government workers launched a virtual mentoring program (http://www.govloop.com) that connected retired civil servants with relatively new public sector professionals who were seeking to move their career to the next level. This virtual government-wide mentoring program not only reaches out across the varying levels of government (federal, state, and local) but also bridges the expanse between agencies, experience, and geographic distance. It now has more than 60,000 members.

Andrew Krzmarzick, the Community Manager Mentors Program coordinator for GovLoop, occasionally offers webinars that give an inside look at the design, development, and delivery of the program, as well as lessons learned. Mentors and mentees who have participated in the program also share how GovLoop's program worked for them. Krzmarzick suggests that successful online mentoring programs require mentors and mentees to exchange emails at least every 2 weeks, that the relationship last at least 3 months (during which there will be at least two formal meetings: face-to-face or on something like Skype or GoToMeeting.com), and that there should be no set content per email or meeting. So today, both formally and informally, mentors and mentees use social media to keep in touch, ask for and give advice, share breaking information, and offer help and assistance.

The American Assembly for Men in Nursing currently has a free-of-charge online pilot mentorship program (http://aamn. org/mentor-program.shtml) adapted from *The Mentor's Guide: Facilitating Effective Learning Relationships* (Zachary, 2000).

NOTE

I have mentored through such mechanisms as Skype, texting, Twitter, and Facebook. I have been mentoring an upcoming leader from Italy for more than 3 years, primarily using Skype, augmented by the occasional email and phone call.

Are There Any "Rules" For Mentors?

Yes, and if followed they can lead to a successfully and mutually beneficial mentor/mentee relationship. Mentors are not only men. Mentees are not only men. Mentorship is not unique to men or to nursing. Good mentoring is good mentoring, in all professions and by either gender. The form it takes is more influenced by the personalities of the mentor and mentee than their genders. It is, by its very nature, generic.

Nursing is not only men. Health care is not only men. If men wish to succeed in nursing and health care, then they will have to acknowledge and embrace the facts. To succeed, men must become integral to the profession. To do this, they must integrate themselves into the profession—and into the various nursing organizations. And yes, those organizations mostly comprise women. As nursing is primarily a woman's profession, this fact should surprise no one. If men want to succeed in nursing—and many men have done so—they must learn to deal with female prejudice against male leadership in nursing, engendered to no small extent by male domination in health care leadership roles.

> **NOTE**
>
> *I personally have been mentored by both men and women. I learned invaluable lessons from my first head nurse and my first director of nursing, both of whom were women. They were tough on me, but I appreciate to this day what they taught me.*

Rule 1: Share a Vision

Clearly, an informal mentor/mentee relationship is both personal and very human. It is also an ongoing relationship that usually but not always develops into a friendship. Therefore, Rule 1 is that a mentor looks for a mentee who shares the same or similar vision of nursing, patients, and the profession as he does. Likewise, the mentee looks for a mentor whose vision and values he shares. Mentoring is not about changing someone's values but rather about fully developing the mentee's possibilities; and it is unlikely that any mentor will willingly devote his time, effort, and passion to someone who doesn't share his vision and values.

NOTE

When I worked in the intensive care unit of a hospital in New Jersey, I noticed that one of the orderlies was paying very close attention to everything I was doing. He was especially interested in how I responded in a crisis and how I dealt with families. It turned out that he was a nursing student who wanted to learn nursing practice from me. He wanted to learn my techniques. I was about the only male nurse with whom he had contact, and he was fascinated. As we spoke, we learned that we shared much the same vision about nursing, and what men could offer the profession. We worked together during his entire undergraduate career. This student went on to become a very successful nurse, and he is currently a chief nursing officer. I recently had the opportunity to see him in action when a relative of mine was admitted to his hospital. I witnessed how highly regarded he was and how he handled crises. It was truly a rewarding sight to see.

Rule 2: Develop, Don't Dominate

This rule deals with the matter of one-upmanship, of being the boss, the leader. People can perform very well if you dominate them, but what gets lost are the spirit, vitality, and joy (and the full participation of the mentee). When one is in a hierarchical relationship (a superior-subordinate relationship), some part of each person closes down. Being a mentor is not about domination, it is about development. So, Rule 2 is that mentorship is all about making someone else powerful.

So when the mentor approaches the mentee, he is inquiring, exploring, and exchanging perspectives. The mentor wants to ask the mentee:

- What does this (or that) imply?
- What does it mean?
- How would you approach this?

The mentor may be an expert in the field, but the mentee is the "expert" on himself, so they are two equals talking something through.

BEGINNING WITH A LETTER

At the beginning of the relationship, one very helpful strategy is to ask the mentee to write a letter to the mentor, dated the next year, about who he will become during that year with the mentor's help, how he will develop his innate talents, what his vision for the profession is, and how he can achieve his place in it. This strategy helps keep the mentor and mentee on point. The mentee keeps the letter, and then the two review it together a year later to see whether they are on point or if, perhaps, the point has changed. The mentee might then write another letter dated the next year and so on. Although I do not think a mentoring relationship can or should be measured, this is one way to ensure that the mentor is not using the relationship to further his own career (as some academics do by having their graduate students research what they [the professors] are interested in rather than pursuing the students' own interests). It also serves as a way to gauge the mentee's growth.

Rule 3: Don't Doubt Your Mentee

Rule 3 applies to all mentors everywhere: "Never doubt the mentee's capacity to accomplish whatever you dream for him" (Zander & Zander, 2000). This implies, of course, that the mentor also has a dream, one in which he sees the potentials within the mentee fully realized and one in which the mentor sees his legacy alive in the future. This is normal, it is human, and it is why it is absolutely critical for the success of the relationship that both mentor and mentee share vision and values from its very beginning.

NOTE

Jack, a student I was mentoring, asked me time and again which nurses made the most money. In return, I would ask him what interested him. He would say "making money." I was beginning to wonder if I was wasting my time with him. I eventually suggested, "If your greatest interest is making money, then why not become a stockbroker?" Finally I said, "Consider what you have to give. Think about your skills—or the skills you would like to acquire. Ask yourself what brings you alive. When you like something, when it piques your interest, you tend to be good at it. When you are good at your work, you devote more time—at lot more, at least 50 to 60 hours a week—to it. If you do this, you are very likely to be successful, and to make more money than average. But perhaps most importantly, you'll be happy." Jack didn't know which specialty he wanted, so I told him to do some research on the subject. In the end, Jack chose to pursue hospice nursing: certainly not the highest paying job in nursing, but for him, the most satisfying.

Rule 4: Fully Invest Yourself

Rule 4 applies equally to mentors and mentees: Throw yourself fully into your life. Now. Right now. Believe in yourself. If you make a mistake, admit it. Do not deny or excuse it. Learn from it, and laugh at yourself. Life (all of it) is to be lived and enjoyed (even the mistakes, when possible). One of the dumbest things I ever did was to go bungee jumping. To this day, I do not know what possessed me to do it. I spent most of the day nauseated as a result. However, I have enjoyed telling and retelling the story. If you can learn to laugh at yourself, and share your mistakes with good humor, you not only become more human to others but you also have a good time telling your story (regardless of whether others learn from it).

> **NOTE**
>
> *Ken came to me as a doctoral student. He wanted to complete his clinical practicum with me. His greatest desire was to learn about management, about teaching, and also about working successfully with people. He had an entrepreneurial spirit, and so do I. So I mentored him—and shared the good, the bad, and the ugly. He learned and grew—and became almost irreplaceable! When he graduated, I hired him, and we worked together for 13 years. He has now gone on to become a very successful nursing academic. We run into each other in professional circles, but I really enjoy reading his articles in professional journals. I know that I helped influence some of his thinking and ideas. Sometimes it pays to pause and reflect on the potential impact of mentoring, as it is the wonderful mentoring moments that will transfer over time and help shape future generations of men in nursing.*

Rule 5: Take Risks

Akin to Rule 4 is Rule 5: Take risks—not foolish risks, but calculated risks that offer enough positive outcomes to warrant them. Take precautions, too (reasonable and sensible ones). Let the mentee see the risks and the precautions. The very nature of risk means that you have a good chance of failing. If you do, discuss the failure (and your fallback plans with the mentee). Make him a part of the process as well as part of the comeback or the successful outcome.

> **NOTE**
>
> *At one point in my career, I was a hospital chief nursing officer. I was successful by anyone's measure. However, I had a dream that somehow we could bring nursing service*

and nursing education together again. So, when a position opened up at the National League for Nursing, I was very interested in applying for it. I asked my colleagues what they thought, and most counseled against it. It would be a step down for me in both title and earning capacity. However, my dream wouldn't go away, and when I talked to my life-long mentor who also was a very successful association executive, he advised me to go for it. Sometimes a mentee takes a risk by following his mentor's advice—and this was risky—but it opened a whole new world for me; I am grateful for it to this day.

Rule 6: Show Mentees What's Possible

A close cousin to Rule 5, Rule 6 holds that a mentor should personify possibility for his mentee. Let him know what you faced and what you overcame. And perhaps most important of all, share with him *how* you overcame an obstacle. In short, let him know you are not Superman; you did not leap over the gender gap in a single bound. Perhaps you'll also want to address how patience, kindness, and (most of all) persistence brought you through. Admit where you failed, what discouraged you, and who and what inspired you. Share your story.

Rule 7: Accept Accountability

Part of sharing your story inevitably leads to Rule 7: Accept accountability. Ordinarily, we equate accountability with guilt and innocence, winners and losers, persecutors and victims. It is to enter the world of "I am right and you are wrong." Or vice versa. It appeals to our instinctive sense of fairness. But remember that however much you may feel a sense of satisfaction or even vindication by blaming (and even proving) that someone else is responsible for your own misfortune, placing yourself in this position portrays you as a loser, perhaps even a poor loser.

So instead of seeking to assign blame, analyze what happened and how you contributed (even if inadvertently or innocently) to the situation so that you can take back a measure of effectiveness, if not even some degree of control over your life and fate. Accept accountability for your life and what occurs in it. It is empowering and liberating, and it completely changes your own attitude and your life. For as you think, so you *are*.

Applying Mentoring to Nursing

These rules apply to any mentoring relationship. But in terms of mentoring in nursing, the American Assembly for Men in Nursing (AAMN) is piloting a mentor program. The philosophy of the AAMN program is based on this premise: "The American Assembly for Men in Nursing (AAMN) Mentor Program promotes the personal and professional achievements of men in nursing through formal and informal collegial relationships while advancing the practice and science of nursing" (http://aamn.org/mentor-program.shtml).

This pilot program involves up to 20 mentor–mentee pairs in its first year. All participants receive printed and electronic resources to assist them as they develop their relationships. In addition, all mentors must complete a brief orientation to become a mentor for the AAMN Mentor Program. The program's structure is adapted from the work of Lois Zachary. In addition to these readings and exercises, the AAMN provides a booklet written by Linda Phillip-Jones titled *The Mentor's Guide* to help mentors facilitate the experience.

Mentoring Groups

Mentoring groups help mentees identify development goals and build the competence necessary to reach them. The primary purpose of most groups is career development, although some might form to expose members to cross-functional and cross-geographic issues (or for many other purposes, ranging from spiritual development to increased social and emotional intelligence). Phillips-Jones defines a mentoring group as

"a collection of mentoring relationships that meets together on a regular basis for an agreed upon length of time. The group's primary purpose is to help mentees accomplish two tasks:

1. Set important development goals and

2. Build competence and character to reach those goals"

(Phillips-Jones, n.d.)

A group usually consists of 8 to 12 mentees and one, two, or three mentor-facilitators. As a result, multiple mentoring relationships develop between the mentees and the mentor-facilitators and among the mentees themselves.

Mentoring groups offer some advantages over one-on-one mentoring:

- An organization can optimize the reach of a normally relatively small group of qualified and willing mentors.

- By working together in a group, mentees may build a valuable network, helping the organization move at a similar pace as the mentees move into positions of greater responsibility.

- These groups also provide more checks and balances because mentees receive multiple sources of feedback.

- The use of group mentoring helps normalize a mentoring culture throughout the organization.

You need to be aware of some disadvantages to group mentoring, as well:

- Mentees do not have as personalized help or one-on-one contact with mentors.

- Rather than a personal relationship, a group or even team relationship may exert pressure on individuals to meet the group's expectations rather than their own.

- Some people do not like to discuss personal performance issues in front of a group of people.

- If people do frankly discuss their issues, expectations, or goals and so forth, the issue of confidentiality arises, which, although an explicit expectation of the groups, may be violated.

People have different perceptions of whether they have helped others—or have been helped by them. The relationship is usually reciprocal in that the mentor may learn as much from the mentee as the mentee learns from him. Indeed, we have all met kind people who have helped us in a variety of ways: counseling, coaching, sponsoring, even teaching us how to survive and prosper, whether in school or in the workplace.

So, what distinguishes *mentoring* from other kinds of assistance? Mentors model behaviors to help mentees see in action the behaviors that will help them reach their goals. Mentees perceive the one helping them as a mentor! In fact, most of us can recall by name the people who have helped us grow and move our careers forward, and we are forever grateful to them.

MEN IN NURSING MENTORING SURVIVAL TIPS

Take advantage of social media mentoring opportunities.

Take the risk of seeking out opportunities in an uncertain world.

Be vigilant because health care reform will open doors for new roles for men as well as new and different practice settings.

Join groups like the American Assembly for Men in Nursing to expand your networking opportunities and rub elbows with men influencing nursing.

Select your mentor carefully. Seek men as mentors who are successful but who also inspire you personally.

Become an active member of mainstream professional groups where men have been successful, such as the American Association of Nurse Anesthetists (AANA), Association of periOperative Registered Nurses (AORN), American Organization of Nurse Executives (AONE), and Sigma Theta Tau International. Men have been elected president of each of these organizations.

Seek mentors beyond our national borders because you can learn much from other men in different cultures.

Be willing to take risk sometimes even when others advise against it.

Be flexible and learn to love change and have the courage to challenge.

Remember that the best "mentor"—and your only life-long mentor—will be the network you develop at work and within professional organizations.

References

Institute of Medicine (IOM). (2010). *The future of nursing: Leading change, advancing health.* Washington, DC: The National Academies Press.

Krzmarzick, A. (2012). Social mentoring: From Telemachus to telecommuters. Retrieved from http://www.govloop.com/profiles/blogs/social-mentoring-from-telemachus-to-telecommuters?elq=2b7e20d6da2142b7a004886ae8ab4d71&elqCampaignId=1954

Phillips-Jones, L. (n.d.). Essentials of mentoring groups, rings, or circles, part 1. Retrieved from http://www.mentoringgroup.com/html/articles/idea_56.htm

Zachary, L. (2000). *The mentor's guide: Facilitating effective learning relationships*. San Francisco, CA: Jossey-Bass.

Zander, R. S., & Zander, B. (2000). *The art of possibility: Transforming professional and personal life*. Watertown, MA: Harvard Business School Press.

Chapter 6

Lack of Racial Diversity in Nursing: An Ongoing Problem Among Men Entering Nursing

Jonathan Lee, BS, RN
UC Davis Medical Center

The experiences of men in nursing are many and varied, with the experiences of those of minority ethnic backgrounds even more so. Therefore, generalizing them all into a standard set of experiences accomplishes little. Although I understand that all minority men in nursing have unique experiences specific to their ethnic heritage and themselves as individuals, dwelling on how experiences differ from one group to another serves only to widen the perceived disparities, which are wide enough already. The only way to neutralize the discrimination and micro-aggressions that minority nurses and nursing students face is to focus on the principles of this profession.

To equip those of you who are minority men entering into or working in nursing, this chapter primarily covers the principles and insights to facilitate your passage through the difficulties you might face during your nursing careers. I respect that I am writing for many of you who might sometimes feel like freaks of nature: males in a female-dominated profession, racial minorities in a profession that is over 80% Caucasian and at least in the United States (U.S. Department of Health and Human Services, Health Resources and Services Administration, 2010). Ultimately, each nurse has to decide whether to make race or ethnicity an issue in his career. Without question, you will face individuals, circumstances, and institutional barriers that will test your commitment to nursing, but it is your responsibility to focus on the principles: We are nurses, and we are here to advance the health of our patients.

Realizing the Need for Racial Diversity Among Men in Nursing

As explained earlier in this book, the nursing profession needs men to increase gender diversity. However, in addition to the need for gender diversity, the profession needs minority male nurses for ethnic and racial diversity. Some, of course, do not consider ethnic and racial diversity a priority in health care, and some who do rarely articulate more than the inherent benefits offered by diversity in any situation. So, why exactly do we need ethnic diversity in the nursing profession?

The answer comes from the diverse patient population of the United States. In 2003, the Institute of Medicine (IOM) published the report *Unequal Treatment*, which found racial and ethnic disparities in health care across a broad spectrum of conditions and services. Some of these disparities result from differences in socioeconomic status and the accessibility of health care in underserved areas (among other things), but the report found that, even after controlling for these factors, racial and ethnic disparities remain.

For instance, the report cites several studies that found that even after controlling for clinical factors such as stage of cancer at diagnosis, significant racial disparities remain in the utilization of appropriate cancer diagnostics and analgesics. In both cancer and cardiovascular disease, differences in care correlate with higher mortality in minority populations. When comparing HIV outcomes, minorities experience lower survival rates, the result of disparities in quality of care even when access to care is comparable. The list of disparities continues through pediatrics, maternal health, mental health, diabetes, end-stage renal disease, kidney transplant, rehabilitation, hospice, and nursing home care. Disparities are seen in the utilization of surgical procedures, as well, either with the underutilization of certain necessary or desirable procedures or in some instances with the increased utilization of less-than-optimal procedures (bilateral orchiectomy, lower limb amputation, and so on). The report's first finding was correspondingly as follows: "Racial and ethnic disparities in healthcare exist and, because they are associated with worse outcomes in many cases, are unacceptable" (IOM, 2003).

After outlining the nature of these disparities, *Unequal Treatment* explores the potential sources of disparities in care. Some evidence suggests patients are one possible source. Racial and ethnic minority patients tend to delay longer before seeking care, decline recommended services, and comply poorly with accepted treatment. This can stem from cultural misunderstandings, miscommunication, negative prior interactions with providers and the health care system, or insufficient knowledge. As noted, though, racial and ethnic variations in patient preferences are small and do not account for the full spectrum and severity of health care disparities.

The report also looks at health systems and how they might influence health care disparities. It cites language barriers as a serious issue, particularly where health systems do not have the means to provide interpreters or translators either in person or through other channels. The report also identifies state government pressure on minorities to enroll in managed care organizations as a risk factor for the displacement of culturally sensitive care providers familiar with the languages and customs of their communities. Some research goes further to indicate that once enrolled in managed care plans, minorities are less likely to use health care services.

IOM RECOMMENDATIONS

The Institute of Medicine's report, Unequal Treatment *(2003), outlined a number of findings and a series of recommendations meant to reduce the racial and ethnic disparities in health care. Some of them include:*

"Finding 1-1: Racial and ethnic disparities in healthcare exist and, because they are associated with worse outcomes in many cases, are unacceptable" (p. 6).

"Recommendation 2-2: Increase healthcare providers' awareness of disparities" (p. 6).

"Finding 3-1: Many sources—including health systems, healthcare providers, patients, and utilization managers— may contribute to racial and ethnic disparities in healthcare" (p. 12).

"Finding 4-1: Bias, stereotyping, prejudice, and clinical uncertainty on the part of healthcare providers may contribute to racial and ethnic disparities in healthcare. While indirect evidence from several lines of research supports this statement, a greater understanding of the prevalence and influence of these processes is needed and should be sought through research" (p. 12).

"Recommendation 5-3: Increase the proportion of underrepresented U.S. racial and ethnic minorities among health professionals" (p. 14).

"Recommendation 5-5: Provide greater resources to the U.S. DHHS Office for Civil Rights to enforce civil rights laws" (p. 15).

"Recommendation 5-6: Promote the consistency and equity of care through the use of evidence-based guidelines" (p. 16).

"Recommendation 5-8: Enhance patient–provider communication and trust by providing financial incentives for practices that reduce barriers and encourage evidence-based practice" (p. 17).

"Recommendation 5-9: Support the use of interpretation services where community need exists" (p. 17).

These findings and recommendations are only a few of those in the full report, but they offer a glimpse of the complexity and difficulty of reducing health care disparities. Some of them rely on large institutions or will take many years more for you or me to see their effects, while others are actionable on the individual level or can begin to help patients on a large scale now. One example of the latter is providing interpretation services where community need exists. In every clinical rotation, I saw at least one example where a language barrier was preventing a patient from getting the care they needed. In some cases, interpretation services were available, and after effective communication, the right care was provided. In other cases, no interpretation was available, and interactions between patients, their families, and providers would become unhelpfully tense, and patients went without the care they really needed.

A significant portion of the report explores patient–provider interactions and the effects that providers have on their patients' care experience and health care disparities. Clinical uncertainty, time pressure, and limited resources, for example, may force many care providers to rely more on easily observable traits (that is, race or ethnicity) rather than on conclusive data gathered from diagnostics or from interacting with the patient, resulting in treatment decisions that might not prove ideal for a patient's needs. Implicit stereotyping by providers, which is not overt or at times even conscious, has also been shown to shape interpersonal interactions and can produce self-fulfilling prophesies during clinical encounters.

Although most health care providers undoubtedly consider prejudice morally objectionable and in conflict with professional standards, many providers may not be aware of how prejudice manifests when interacting with patients, as suggested by research where a patient's race or ethnicity was found to have influenced his or her provider's diagnostic conclusion, treatment prescription, and feelings regarding the patient.

On the patient side, minority patients do perceive greater racial discrimination in health care. This is associated with patient mistrust and refusal or poor compliance with treatment, which may in turn influence provider investment in the care process. The report finds that patient and provider attitudes influence each other in turn, but adds that the care provider is significantly more powerful during clinical encounters than the patient, making the provider an important focus for intervention.

Accordingly, Recommendation 5-3 of the report, as noted earlier in the chapter, is as follows: "Increase the proportion of underrepresented U.S. racial and ethnic minorities among health professionals" (IOM, 2003). As justification, the report cites the improved patient participation, satisfaction, and care compliance associated with patient–provider relationships strengthened by racial concordance and the fact that minority providers are more likely to serve in medically underserved areas. Based on this information, health care has need for racial and ethnic minority providers familiar with the language, customs, and values of minority patients. To that end, the nursing profession needs racial and ethnic minority nurses as well as male nurses, and that's where minority male nurses come in.

Facing the Issues of Minority Men in Nursing

Whether you are considering nursing, are in nursing school, or are working as a nurse already, as a minority you will face numerous challenges in the profession by virtue of your minority status. These challenges often involve financial or academic stresses or involve issues of emotional support. These three categories do not encompass all the issues that men in nursing have faced throughout history and will face in the future, but they do provide some context for how to focus on and apply principles, especially when under stress.

Financial Issues

If you are considering nursing, are in nursing school, or are thinking about returning to nursing school, a key element you must consider is how to pay for your nursing education. Nursing school, like any other professional education, is expensive for anyone, and for many ethnic and racial minorities, paying for it can prove to be a real burden. One could write several books just on paying for nursing school, but because that's beyond the scope of this chapter, I limit this to a review of possible strategies.

As with paying for any type of higher education, paying for nursing school might require you to take out loans, apply for scholarships and grants, or work one or more jobs to make ends meet while you pursue your education. Depending on your financial situation and circumstances, you may need to rely on one of these strategies or combine a few that work for you:

- At the nursing school I attended, many of my class-mates in the undergraduate prelicensure program took out loans from the school to make up the difference between expenses and what they could pay, many qualified for or won scholarships from the school or the adjacent health system, and many worked as nursing assistants or unit secretaries or else did a combination of the three to pay their way through.

- Some who were returning to nursing school for a career change relied on savings they accumulated in their previous career. Tuition-assistance programs from the institutions they worked at aided some who were already nurses and were returning for advanced degrees.

- Other institutions offer loan-repayment programs.

- Many states also offer scholarships for those willing to work in medically underserved areas for a set number of years, something that may appeal to you as a minority health professional.

Again, which of these strategies you choose depends largely on what works for you, your family, and your situation.

However, I do want to expand on working while in nursing school because of the significant additional burdens it places on you as an individual. As someone who worked several part-time jobs during my nursing education, I would frame this option as a high-risk, high-return strategy. Should you choose to work while in nursing school, be aware that nursing school is not easy as it is and to balance work while excelling in class and clinical rotations demands exceptional time-management skills, balance, and tenacity, as well as support from those around you. Even with these elements, the risk of burnout increases with the number of hours you work each week, the nature of your work, the nature of the course material and load during a term, and long clinical hours. And that doesn't even take into account the need for extracurricular activities and a supportive social life. Balancing all these aspects of your life and maintaining activity and excellence in each of them is difficult. Often, one aspect or another will take up more and more of your time and resources to the detriment of the other aspects. When that happens, you might find it exceedingly difficult to bring your life back into balance.

MAINTAINING BALANCE

You've probably seen tips all over the place about how to maintain work-life balance. I am no self-help counselor or work-life balance expert, but here are a few things that I found helpful to keep my life in relative balance.

- **Find a constructive hobby (or hobbies) that you enjoy:** *For me, it was martial arts and music. Being able to spend a day each week to train in the martial arts and do something totally different from class and clinical was an enormous relief. Being able to play the piano or guitar for a half hour after class or on a day off helped me to unwind and just enjoy the music. I also think that it helped me to stop hearing alarm monitors when I wasn't in the hospital.*

- **Stay active:** *I know that oftentimes after back-to-back 12-hour shifts, class, and whatever other commitments you might have, you get home and you just want to do nothing or sleep. In the mornings before class or clinical, you just want to get there on time. During a shift, you may feel yourself nodding off. When you can,*

continues

go for a jog; even a walk after work can help.
Take a yoga class on your days off, or go to the
gym with a friend. Do some warm-up exercises
before going to class or clinical, walk or bike to
where you need to be, or take the stairs up to
your class or floor. If you're falling asleep during
a shift, stand up, move around, do some squats,
or go for a walk during your break. Staying
active is crucial to countering fatigue and helps
with maintaining focus.

- **Talk to people:** *Balancing everything is hard,*
  and sometimes it feels like other people just
  don't get it. People don't always want to get it,
  but if they want to, helping them to understand
  what you are going through might help you, too.
  Sometimes it doesn't take much to help someone
  understand, and sometimes you just need that
  someone to understand. Still, if for whatever
  reason your personal support structure just isn't
  in a position to understand when you need it to,
  see if you have options for counseling or therapy.
  In my senior year, my entire class was exhausted,
  and no one was really in any position to lend a
  listening ear. I was fortunate to have affordable
  access to the school's counseling services as well
  as a good counselor who was able to help me
  through some difficult times.

Even so, working during nursing school can provide many
opportunities. In addition to a measure of financial stability and
a feeling of self-worth, certain kinds of employment offer distinct
advantages. Working in a health care setting, for instance,
offers the chance to become familiar with health insurance,
documentation systems, patient interactions, and nursing
procedures, to name a few things. In addition, if the institution

where you work also happens to be hiring nurses when you graduate from nursing school, you often have a better chance of getting the job by virtue of your internal applicant status.

Even if you do not find part-time employment where you plan to work as a nurse (for example, a medical center, community hospital, or nursing home), many types of employment offer opportunities to develop skills that apply to your nursing career. Many of my classmates worked as babysitters or home-health aides, which developed their ability to interact with pediatric and geriatric patient populations, respectively. I worked as a technology consultant and then as a technology supervisor for students at my institution. In both positions, I had the opportunity to acquire unique skills with a broad range of current technology, teach technical workshops, train employees, and manage staffing. The principles for building technical proficiency, teaching theory and application, and managing a system readily apply to nursing. As an assistant instructor for martial arts, I taught classes of different sizes and skill levels and developed the same awareness and teaching skills that all nurses use on a daily basis. As a mentor for the National Council on Aging's Better Choices, Better Health program, I interacted with patients online and studied chronic disease processes and self-management skills that are valuable to anyone. In each realm of employment, I also found close friends and valuable professional connections.

As a minority male nurse, I would especially encourage you to consider jobs where you regularly interact with people other than your colleagues. Customer service and teaching are two broad categories that come to mind. Gender and cultural awareness and sensitivity go both ways, and interacting with people who think, learn, and communicate differently can help you to examine your own perspectives and beliefs and develop an understanding of someone who is different from you. This understanding can give you a significant advantage in your daily interactions with others as well as when you are faced with intolerance. Of course, if you have trouble finding a customer service or teaching job, you need not worry. Regardless of what job you get, the opportunities to develop skills and connections in the employment you find are limited only by your attitude and imagination. You can make your job work for you.

> **NOTE**
>
> *As a caveat, though, I want to add that it was not wise for me to have worked all three of the previously mentioned part-time jobs concurrently while being the president of two moderate-sized campus organizations. Those jobs and activities on top of classes and clinicals and some other issues resulted in my burnout during my last year of nursing school, and I only recovered in time to graduate with my cohort thanks to the support of some very understanding superiors, faculty, and friends. Being employed while pursuing your nursing education can provide valuable returns and opportunities, but know yourself, your limits, and how to take care of yourself. It's been said before ad nauseum, but it is particularly important for nurses: You cannot take care of other people if you cannot take care of yourself.*

Academic Issues

After you have the financial aspect figured out, as much as practical at least, turn your attention to the academic aspect of nursing and nursing education. To reiterate, as a professional school, nursing school is not easy for anyone, and it can be downright hard if you are not accustomed to the academic rigor. As nursing advances as a profession, more and more emphasis is placed on the science and the research that makes the best nursing care possible. In the clinical setting, quality nursing care requires knowledge of chemistry, math, physics, physiology, pathophysiology, pharmacology, and psychology in addition to languages, communication and cultural studies, and history. Proficiency at such a broad spectrum of subjects and the constant updating of knowledge in each discipline are traits that define the nursing profession and have created a culture of lifelong learning. The rigor of such an academic environment is demanding, but now more than ever, the nursing profession needs smart, hardworking, and talented individuals like you to succeed in nursing and move the profession forward.

Emotional Issues

Before you roll your eyes at the idea of manly men having emotional issues, let me remind you that, like it or not, men do have emotions. What's more, compassion is a requisite for nursing, and compassion is an emotion. Many of you may have felt firsthand what it is like to have friends or family in the hospital; indeed, feeling those emotions may be part of the reason you are considering nursing. These emotions are like those experienced by nurses at the bedside; after all, nurses are human, too.

Nursing is an emotionally trying profession. Having to address, communicate, and interact with multiple patients, their families, other care providers, and support personnel while human lives depend on you, all while your own personal life goes on, is stressful, to say the least. As a minority male who desires to excel in your professional education and career and a host of commitments on top of them, nursing can push you further than you've ever gone or believed you could go. From the tension and responsibility of day-to-day care, to the outrage at injustice, to the passion of advocacy, to the delight of seeing life renewed, to the sorrow that comes with the loss of life, you need support throughout your nursing education and career. This help can come from many places, whether from family or friends, classmates or coworkers, instructors or mentors, or even pets or your own patients, but you do need it.

Overcoming an Unwillingness to Ask for Help

In dealing with the issues outlined earlier, having help can make your life a lot easier. But if you are like many men, regardless of whether they are in nursing, you exhibit a general unwillingness to ask for help. For ethnic and racial minority males, cultural norms and perceived pressure from minority and majority groups often reinforce the unwillingness to ask for help. If you are one of those who can ask for help at the right time and in the right way, I am relieved. For those who are not, I will try to explain why you need to learn how.

Nursing is a challenging profession, if you have not figured that out already, and you will need support in nursing school and in the nursing profession. Whether it is financial, academic, emotional, or some other kind of support, you will need it in your nursing career. Even if you are the most capable, self-sufficient, and independent individual alive, you will need support. Nursing is a demanding and collaborative profession where people in a group support each other in meeting the needs of the population. It is not a profession for islands.

If you can accept that you need help, you must next answer this: What prevents you from asking for it? The reasons are probably infinite, but in the spirit of focusing on principles, let me just say that asking for help when you need it does not reflect poorly on your character. Indeed, it is more often a sign of strength and determination, and the help you receive simply from asking for it may move you forward on the path to a successful nursing career.

However, some of you might have asked for help and found none or even had people try to hurt your education or career; this will sound hollow to you, but all is not lost. If you have tried everything you can possibly think of and then some without success, maintain a positive attitude and focus on your principles. Do not lose faith or hope in yourself or your chosen profession. It is unquestionably much easier for me to say this than for anyone, including myself, to actually do, especially when you feel that you have nowhere to turn. In my experience, though, help often comes from the most unlikely of places at the least likely of times.

SEEKING HELP FROM PROFESSIONAL ORGANIZATIONS

One resource that can provide you with options should you need help is a professional organization for any kind of minority group in nursing. The American Assembly for Men in Nursing (AAMN) is one such organization for men in nursing. The various associations under the National Coalition of Ethnic and Minority Nurse Associations represent other options for minority nurses, as the name suggests. As with all national professional organizations, they provide a wide range of resources, professional connections, and career opportunities that may be what you need to get back on track.

Dealing with Identity Issues

As an ethnic minority male in nursing, you may find your identity tested throughout your life. In the academic or clinical setting, you may encounter tension between your ethnic identity and those of other ethnic identities, whether they are majority or minority identities. This tension, combined with the seemingly contradictory demands placed on your own ethnic identity, especially in a multiethnic nation like the United States, can make it easy to fall prey to the seemingly inevitable cycle of interracial conflict. Unfortunately, should you fall into this cycle, you will only hinder everything you hope to achieve. Because you are reading this, though, I believe that you are one who can and will come to terms with your own identity and rise above the cycle of interracial tension and conflict. In your daily life and career, strive to focus on principles: You are a nurse, and you are here to advance the health of patients. To help you on this path when things gets rough—and they undoubtedly will—I give you the words of John Watson. Although he says *man*, Watson's words apply to anyone (Watson, 1903):

> "*This man beside us also has a hard fight with an unfavouring world, with strong temptations, with doubts and fears, with wounds of the past which have skinned over, but which smart when they are touched. It is a fact, however surprising. And when this occurs to us we are moved to deal kindly with him, to bid him be of good cheer, to let him understand that we are also fighting a battle; we are bound not to irritate him, nor press hardly upon him nor help his lower self.*" (p. 168-169)

My hope is that this quote from Watson will be a gentle reminder that you are human and so is everyone around you. Everyone is shaped by their experiences and influenced by those around them, and in the midst of difficult lives, some have not learned that sexism and racism are not acceptable ways to convey their feelings or experiences. This is not to excuse those individuals. Without question, no one ever has a right to use gender or ethnicity as a way to vent their negative emotions, but no one's negativity has a right to affect you either. I don't think it has ever been easy to shrug off discrimination and prejudice, but I hope this reminder will help to keep that from happening.

Overcoming Barriers to Clinical Experiences

Unfortunately, you will find some institutions that simply do not trust male nurses or minority nurses. As minority male nurses, you may find yourself a target of this mistrust. In your education and career, you may meet or perhaps have already met some patients who simply do not want a male nurse, sometimes even more so a minority male nurse. At most institutions, a different nurse will be assigned to meet patient preferences. You may experience discrimination from others in the clinical setting by virtue of your gender, ethnicity, or both. By any standard, such discrimination is difficult to contend with. When all you are trying to do is make the most of a possible learning experience or help someone in need, encountering discrimination can take a toll on your confidence in the nursing profession. The simple injustice of it is disgraceful, and injustice has a way of triggering any range of emotions in all of us, few of them constructive.

But when faced with such behavior, your own behavior is all the more influential. You want to be a nurse who rises above prejudice and bigotry by focusing on the principles. You are a professional nurse: competent, reliable, and dedicated. You are there to advance the health of your patients, whoever they may be. Your ethnic heritage and gender are irrelevant. All that matters is your ability to fulfill your duty as a nurse. Consider this and ask yourself whether you will let someone's intolerance control your behavior to the detriment of all or if you will use your principles to influence the behavior of others and bring about healing.

FINDING COMMON GROUND

To help you with this, you can try this whenever you feel isolated or discriminated against in the face of a majority population: Remember that most people are the same. You do not differ so much from other people, just as they do not differ so much from you. Consider commonalities between you and those around you. For example, if you are in nursing school, even if you are the only ethnic minority man in a class of Caucasian women, everyone

continues

probably feels just as nervous on the first day of clinical. Maybe some of them share your interest in perioperative nursing. Once you can identify the commonalities between yourself and others, you can begin to see the nuances between those in the majority. Even those of the same ethnic heritage and gender have differences among them. Some may be passionate about pediatrics, whereas others can't imagine being anywhere except geriatrics. Some may go running every day after class, while others prefer yoga or dance. Being able to identify how similar you are to those around you and appreciate the nuances that make everyone different means that being of a different gender and ethnic heritage matters much less than others might try to make you believe.

The only time your ethnic heritage might matter is when it has the potential to improve a patient's experience. As mentioned earlier in this chapter, some patients feel more comfortable or comply more readily with treatment when their provider shares the same race as them. If at any point an interaction surrounding race begins to takes a negative slant, bring it back to basics and remember to keep it professional: You are their nurse.

Issues for Institutions When Recruiting and Retaining Men in Nursing

Like individuals in nursing, institutions have to deal with issues of diversity when they seek to recruit and retain men in nursing. As mentioned earlier in this chapter, racial and ethnic diversity in all health care professions is central to the health of a population. If you are responsible for recruitment and retention, the importance of recruiting and retaining minority men in nursing is evidence based. As with the issues faced by men in nursing, the issues faced by institutions seeking to recruit and retain them cannot all be mentioned here. Therefore, I discuss only some of the issues and strategies that you may want to consider in your institution's quest for a diverse and adaptable nursing staff.

Recruitment Stage

During the recruiting process, you can draw prospective recruits' interest if they perceive that your institution not only has diversity but is also committed to it. Your institution can demonstrate their diversity through indirect communication and through in-person contact with potential recruits.

For indirect communication, several elements can make minority male recruits more comfortable. In recruiting media such as informational pamphlets, program brochures, or residency advertisements, show a balance of all ethnicities and genders (ideally both genders of every ethnicity would be shown) and present them in comparable roles and postures. On websites, feature pictures and articles with accomplished students of a variety of genders and ethnicities. Be advised that with any kind of recruiting media you may discover fine lines between highlighting diversity and undervaluing the accomplishments of nonminorities, changing the public perception of nursing and reinforcing current attitudes, providing transparency on the current reality, or presenting a vision of what things should be. Decisions about recruiting materials should, accordingly, be the subject of extensive, sound, and well-reasoned discussion to see what aligns most closely with your institution's mission and values.

In addition to showcasing the diversity of your institution's students and staff, other elements can positively affect the recruitment of minorities. A diversity clause included as part of your institution's values or mission statement is one example. As a follow-up to that, ask applicants on their applications or during interviews "How are you different?" and "How can you add to the diversity of this organization?" Combining these two elements shows a definitive commitment to supporting diversity at your institution and can go a long way toward reaching out to minority men in nursing.

DIVERSITY CLAUSES AND STATEMENTS

A public commitment to diversity can go a long way in recruitment, and having a diversity clause can be as simple as including it in a list of values:

Our values are Respect, Excellence, Accountability, Diversity, Compassion, and Teamwork

A more developed example would be a statement such as:

Diversity—We encourage and celebrate the diversity of experiences, beliefs, values, needs, and expectations of our patients, providers, and staff.

If it fits with your institutional aims, I would encourage you to consider having not just a diversity clause, but a complete diversity statement. One example would be the University of Washington School of Nursing's Diversity Statement:

> *"A fundamental purpose of nursing is the provision of quality and equitable health care to all members, groups, and communities of society. Nursing knowledge and practice must be sufficiently broad in perspective and content to meet the requirements of a diverse, multicultural population. To this end, the University of Washington School of Nursing seeks to attract, admit/hire, and support diverse and racially repre- sentative students, staff, and faculty members.*

> *A central activity to support this diverse community is adequate preparation to interact with people from all cultures. This focus requires that nursing be responsive*

to, explicitly value, and incorporate a wide variety of perspectives and experiences. This open and flexible approach is based on respect for all cultures and their members, on examination of our own perspectives, biases, and socialization, and on the ability to examine and adjust our own perspectives, beliefs, and behaviors.

We are committed to fostering a climate that is inclusive and welcoming of all groups. We recognize that this effort is a multi-dimensional one that includes: recruitment efforts, policies, curriculum, pedagogy, norms, practices, faculty/staff promotions, decision making, and continuing multicultural and anti-oppression education for faculty and staff members. We also recognize that nursing education and practice in the United States occurs within the social, cultural, and historical context of institutionalized racism (among other forms of oppression). Meeting our purpose thus requires a sustained and multi-dimensional effort.

We are committed to eliminating all forms of oppression resulting from socially and culturally constructed differences in race/ethnicity, sex/gender identity or orientation, socioeconomic status, language, age, physical characteristics, disability, pregnancy, veteran status, country of origin, citizenship, religious or political beliefs, military status, and others.

UW School of Nursing Principles of Inclusion

1. *We affirm the inherent dignity of each individual and group.*

2. *We affirm that group differences are socially, culturally, and historically constructed and hierarchically arranged, resulting in the inequitable distribution of resources among groups. This construction and distribution can be changed and we commit to change it.*

continues

3. *We affirm our commitment to address difference, privilege, and power at the School of Nursing. We will address privilege and power using anti-racist and anti-oppression principles of on-going education, open dialogue, skill building, challenging the status quo, and accountability to people of color and other social groups.*

4. *We affirm our commitment to increase the numbers of faculty, students, and staff from underrepresented groups, and to support their leadership within the school.*

5. *We affirm our commitment to work toward a climate of inclusiveness on all levels of the School of Nursing." (University of Washington, School of Nursing, 2001, reprinted with permission)*

Consider what option is most appropriate for your institution.

When recruiting in person, faculty or administrator diversity may be an issue for some potential recruits. Without minority male faculty/administrators, it is easy for minority male applicants to feel less comfortable with the support and power structure presented by the institution. This is not, of course, entirely the fault of institutions. While a complete discourse is beyond the scope of this chapter, with the few minority male nurses to begin with, and with the general scarcity of nurses with the advanced degrees to be faculty or administrators, not many minority male faculty or administrators are available to go around. What's more, although minority male students and staff may identify more readily with minority male faculty and administrators, this most certainly does not preclude other faculty and administrators from connecting with them and acting as excellent role models.

Another element that can make a real difference with the recruitment of minority men in nursing is the presence of support groups. For men in nursing, having an institutional chapter of the AAMN can be a real benefit of being at your institution. For racial and ethnic minority nurses, being part of an association under the National Coalition of Ethnic Minority Nurse Associations (NCEMNA) can also provide support, resources, and opportunities. In addition, having students and nurses who are part of these groups and can speak to the supportive environment of your institution during recruiting events cannot be overstated. The experiences of peers resonate with individuals in ways that other experiences simply cannot.

Retention Stage

After nurses have been recruited, the retention stage is where the institution makes them feel that they are a welcome and valuable part of the team every time they come to work. Like any type of behavioral change, this takes substantial effort from the parties involved. Accordingly, cross-cultural and social justice training should be mandatory for all students, faculty, staff, and administrators. Diversity is a culture unto itself, and it must be maintained by everyone at your institution. In this day and age, implicit stereotypes, unconscious biases, and casual remarks can cause just as much damage to an inclusive environment and are as widespread as overt discrimination once was. It is everyone's responsibility to keep the professional environment professional.

On a related note, clear standards and equal opportunities for success and advancement must be in place at your institution. Be mindful of how minorities perceive these standards and opportunities. Whether in an academic or clinical setting, having a level playing field is vital to retention, supports diversity, and maintains a team's cohesion. Your institution also stands to gain from capitalizing on the cultural perspectives of minority male nurses. Their ability to understand minority patient populations and view situations through their unique experiences can enhance the care provided at your institution.

In addition to having support groups like AAMN or NCEMNA at your institution, actively promote and develop these organizations. Encouraging individuals to join these groups, make use of their services, and take advantage of the opportunities they provide serves not only to retain minority men in nursing but also to enhance the collaboration between these groups and your institution, to the benefit of all involved. Your institution will have the opportunity to showcase your students and staff who are involved with these national organizations, the organization will have accomplished leaders and valuable sponsorship, and both parties receive positive publicity.

CAUTION

One word of caution, though, regarding the development of support groups: Although the support and encouragement of diversity is crucial and beneficial to all, ensure that it is not taken to a level where reverse discrimination and prejudice begin to show themselves. The negative effects of such a development are obvious and difficult to reverse.

Institutions need to celebrate diversity. If differences are noted, they must be celebrated! At the institutional level, the celebration of differences allows people to recognize them and view them in a positive light rather than as ways to label or cast aspersions on any group. When combined with sound recruitment and retention strategies, this has the potential to make your institution more inclusive, progressive, and adaptable to help you to provide the best care experience to your patients and meet their ever-changing needs.

Ultimately, minority males in nursing face difficulty. You will encounter many challenges not only because of your gender but also because of your racial/ethnic heritage. But these challenges also present you with great opportunity: It is time for you as minority men to do your part to advance the nursing profession.

MINORITY MEN IN NURSING SURVIVAL TIPS

As minority men in nursing, you should:

- *Recognize and convey the value that you bring to nursing.*

- *Find a balance between work, school, and personal life.*

- *Plan and prepare for the financial, academic, and emotional demands of a nursing education and the nursing profession.*

- *Learn to ask for help.*

- *Build support networks of family, friends, colleagues, instructors, and/or other professionals.*

- *Remember that everyone is human, including you, your patients, and your colleagues.*

- *Take the opportunity to lead and advance the health of your patients and the nursing profession.*

Nursing institutions should:

- *Ensure that recruitment media portrays diversity.*

- *Make a public commitment to diversity in their missions, visions, and values, and demonstrate it throughout the recruitment process.*

- *Support the development of professional nursing support groups.*

- *Develop and implement a curriculum for universal cross-cultural and social justice training.*

- *Maintain clear standards and equal opportunities.*

- *Celebrate diversity!*

References

Institute of Medicine (IOM). (2003). *Unequal treatment: Confronting racial and ethnic disparities in health care* (full printed version). (B. D. Smedley, A. Y. Stith, & A. R. Nelson, Eds.). Washington, DC: The National Academies Press. Retrieved from http://www.nap.edu/openbook.php?record_id=10260

University of Washington, School of Nursing. (2001). Diversity statement. Retrieved from http://nursing.uw.edu/about/diversity/diversity.html

U.S. Department of Health and Human Services, Health Resources and Services Administration. (2010). The registered nurse population: Findings from the 2008 national sample survey of registered nurses. Retrieved from http://bhpr.hrsa.gov/healthworkforce/rnsurveys/rnsurveyfinal.pdf

Watson, J. (1903). *The homely virtues.* London: Hodder & Stoughton.

Chapter 7
Strengthening the Male Nursing Workforce

Paul J. Larson, MS, RN
Department of Medical Education
Gundersen Lutheran Medical Foundation
La Crosse, Wisconsin

Any plan to strengthen the male nursing workforce must be sustainable, practical, and appealing. One framework of a plan that incorporates these concepts requires a brief history lesson about Caesar and the Roman Empire. Under Caesar's direction, a Roman Empire architect named Vitruvius (see Leonardo Da Vinci's depiction in Figure 7.1) was charged with incorporating the concepts of durability, usefulness, and beauty into each structure he designed and built. Building these structures, some of which still stand today, took hundreds of years and included calculated, systematic planning. Any effective plan to strengthen the male nursing workforce will likewise incorporate the Vitruvian concepts of durability, usefulness, and beauty.

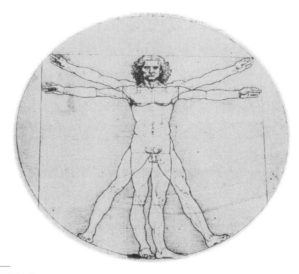

FIGURE 7.1

Leonardo Da Vinci's Vitruvian Man

This chapter outlines sustainable (durable), practical (useful), and appealing (beautiful) steps that nurses, health care organizations, schools, professional organizations, nurse leaders, the media, and others can take to strengthen the male nursing workforce.

The male nursing workforce is small: Approximately 7% of nurses are men (American Association of Colleges of Nursing [AAACN], 2012). The Institute of Medicine (IOM) in *The Future of Nursing: Leading Change, Advancing Health Report Recommendations* notes that efforts to strengthen nursing "should take into consideration strategies to increase the diversity of the nursing workforce in terms of race/ethnicity, gender, and geographic distribution" (IOM, 2010b, p. 4). The IOM's recognition of the need for more gender diversity in nursing and the enormous statistical gender disparity are compelling reasons to attract more men to the field. Acknowledging and accepting this need is easy; however, acting to address the need is challenging and requires steps that must be sustained for generations.

> **NOTE**
>
> *Although it is important for men to be strong advocates for men in nursing, it is also important for our female colleagues to stand beside us as we work together to strengthen the profession. Future use of the terms nurse and nurses in this chapter is intended to be inclusive of all nurses (men and women), but will, no doubt, hold special significance for men.*

Change: Moving Forward from the 7%

The health care industry has tacitly acknowledged the need for more men in nursing for years. Despite this acknowledgement, the proportion of men in nursing has remained relatively unchanged for decades. The word *change* often carries a negative connotation. And yes, change can be arduous, unwelcome, and painful, but it can also be satisfying, desirable, and refreshing.

Knowledge of change and change theory is valuable in designing a sustainable, practical, and appealing plan to strengthen the male nursing workforce. Change experts and theorists and plans abound, and Kotter's eight-stage process of creating major change (Kotter, 1996) is a useful tool to identify past challenges and to provide a fresh approach to the problem.

A Framework for Change

Dr. John Kotter is a former professor at Harvard Business School, a world-renowned change expert, and author of *Leading Change* (1996). His eight-step approach to leading change provides a framework for strengthening the male nursing workforce. Kotter proposed the following eight-stage process to create major change:

1. **Establish a sense of urgency.** The small male nursing workforce, predicted shortage of nurses, and the IOM's recognition of the need to address gender disparity in nursing are separate and distinct recognitions of the need for change. Collectively, they establish a sense of urgency.

2. **Create the guiding coalition.** Creating a group to lead the change is the second step of Kotter's change process. Although individual efforts to facilitate change are welcome and needed, a group that has the power to lead and effect change is a necessary component of a sustainable plan. The group best suited to lead a guiding coalition for change is the American Assembly for Men in Nursing (AAMN), a national organization with leaders and chapters located throughout the country. The AAMN is equipped to lead this change, and its objectives and strategic plan align perfectly with the first step of Kotter's eight-stage process (establish a sense of urgency).

> **NOTE**
>
> *The AAMN objectives (listed in this note) and goal six of its strategic plan (develop strategic relationships to promote the organization, recruitment, and retention of men in nursing and men's health) are clear and directly aimed at strengthening the male nursing workforce (AAMN, 2011; 2013):*
>
> - *Encourage men of all ages to become nurses and join together with all nurses in strengthening and humanizing health care.*

- *Support men who are nurses to grow professionally and demonstrate to each other and to society the increasing contributions being made by men within the nursing profession.*

- *Advocate for continued research, education, and dissemination of information about men's health issues, men in nursing, and nursing knowledge at the local and national levels.*

- *Support members' full participation in the nursing profession and its organizations, and use this Assembly for the limited objectives stated above.*

3. **Develop a vision and strategy.** The AAMN objectives and components of its strategic plan are bullish on men in nursing, and the AAMN has a vision of what the nursing workforce could look like.

4. **Communicate the change vision.** To communicate the vision of what the nursing workforce could look like, the voices of nurses, schools, health care and professional organizations, and the media are necessary. Fortunately, the AAMN's rich web of professional connections is poised to bring them all together in a strong, collective voice for change.

5. **Empower broad-based action.** In this stage, we want to eliminate obstacles, change systems/structures that undermine change, and employ nontraditional ideas and activities. Misconceptions of the nursing profession and stereotypes of male nurses exist and persist. Transforming misconceptions and stereotypes will take sustained broad-based action, including risk taking and innovative ideas. Nurses, health care organizations, middle schools, high schools, colleges, schools of nursing, national advisory organizations

(such as the IOM), professional organizations such as the American Nurses Association (ANA) and the AAMN, and the media all play important roles in empowering broad-based action, as described later in this chapter.

6. **Generate short-term wins.** In this stage, improvements in performance are recognized. For example, a health care organization might recognize a high-achieving male nurse with an employee recognition award; a high school could applaud a graduating senior who receives a scholarship to a school of nursing; or the media could feature a story that includes a male nurse, cover a story about an increase in enrollment of male nursing students, or highlight the number of male nurses in their local health care organizations.

7. **Consolidate gains and produce more change.** As part of this step, nurses, health care organizations, schools, national advisory organizations, professional organizations, and the media communicate their successes. Local and national leaders reaffirm their commitment to maintaining the sense of urgency. When a win is achieved and the male nursing workforce strengthened, the win needs to be celebrated within a unit, department, or organization.

8. **Anchor new approaches in the culture.** As the unit, department, or organization celebrates a strengthened male nursing workforce, all involved must anchor plans for sustaining it.

No one approach to change will work in all environments. For that reason, change theory is valuable because it provides a framework for a plan and a tool for measuring progress and success in organizations of all kinds.

The Power of One: Attracting Men to Nursing

Local, regional, and national efforts to attract men to the nursing profession are necessary, but the foundation of any plan to strengthen the profession begins with the power of one nurse and extends to include programs and organizations that are up to the task. After all, one nurse has profound power to influence others.

Nursing is a high-profile profession, and nurses are responsible for being its good stewards. Stewardship in nursing is important and involves representing and sharing the unique work and life experiences of nursing. Every nurse will have planned and unplanned opportunities to showcase his or her stewardship for the profession. Whatever the setting or opportunity, every nurse has the responsibility to incorporate the concept of stewardship into practice.

Showcasing Stewardship

Opportunities to showcase stewardship abound. Whether at a social gathering, ball game, or a take-your-parent-to-school day, we have many opportunities to share information about our profession. You might face such common questions as, "Why did you choose nursing?" And for men, "Why do you work in a profession in which the vast majority are women?" The answers we provide to these important questions can have profound impact and influence upon an audience of one or of many.

The times and places that nurses encounter these types of questions may be planned or spur of the moment, but every nurse needs to have thoughtful, well-prepared answers.

Some of the best answers come in the form of an "elevator speech"—that is, a well-prepared, brief (approximately 30 seconds, simple response designed to answer the question by informing, engaging, and influencing the audience. Although each nurse will answer these questions differently, all should seize the opportunity to clear up misconceptions and to educate the public about their profession.

NOTE

Paul Hoch, RN, intensive care unit, stated, "Nursing allows me to help others while providing job security, mobility, access to cutting-edge technology, competitive earnings, and a schedule that fits my life. Nursing touches everyone from prenatal care to hospice care and everyone in between. As a nurse, there's no place I can't go. The whole gender issue in nursing has never bothered me. We're all here for the same purpose and all working towards the same goal."

Role Modeling

A powerful way that men and women in nursing can influence others is by being a positive role model. If imitation is the sincerest form of flattery, then role modeling can be a simple but effective tool that all nurses can use to strengthen the profession.

The ANA's *Code of Ethics for Nurses* (2012) describes how each nurse has the responsibility for "carrying out nursing responsibilities in a manner consistent with quality in nursing care and the ethical obligations of the profession." The *Code of Ethics* also describes how terms like *respect, collaboration, accountability, professional growth, integrity, competence,* and *wholeness of character* are important for every nurse to incorporate into his or her practice.

While evidence of these qualities can be found in interactions with patients or colleagues, it can also be found in a nurse's professional memberships, professional publications, attire, and in social settings and interactions in their community. In a church group, coaching a ball game, working on a community fundraiser, or simply speaking and interacting with a family member, friend, neighbor, or stranger, nurses have numerous opportunities to showcase their professionalism and to display the qualities of a respected role model. "For the professional, his or her work is not simply a job. It is, instead, an expression of his or her identity, a representation of his or her ownership of the work and life of the profession that operates at all times and in all places" (Porter-O'Grady & Malloch, 2013, p. 4).

Strong Leaders

The IOM's Report Brief for *The Future Of Nursing: Leading Change, Advancing Health* (2010a) outlines the importance of leadership roles for nurses and states that "all nurses must take responsibility for their personal and professional growth by developing leadership competencies and exercising these competencies across all care settings" (p. 3). Accepted definitions and types of leadership abound, but common leadership-related competencies include qualities such as strength of character, integrity, trust, knowledge, flexibility, creativity, commitment, listening, sensitivity, followership, vision, inspiration, servanthood, and many more. With a patient, on a work-related committee, and in community or social settings, nurses have abundant opportunities to display their leadership skills. Respected male nurse *leaders* are fine examples of strong, high-achieving nurses who lead and invigorate the male nursing workforce.

> **LUTHER CHRISTMAN**
>
> *Luther Christman, PhD, RN, was a legendary nursing pioneer and an outspoken advocate of affirmative action to recruit more men and minorities into the nursing profession. As a young man in World War II, he tried to enlist in the U.S. Army Nurse Corps, but was denied because of his gender. In the years to come he would tell many more stories about how his path to nursing school and the profession was often blocked by women and a nursing culture that discriminated against men. Undeterred, he went on to become the first male dean of a nursing school in the United States, and one of the most honored nurses in the history of nursing.*

> **NOTE**
>
> *In the workplace or in the community, every nurse has a professional responsibility to be a good role model and leader. Perhaps Porter-O'Grady and Malloch (2013) said it best: "For a professional, personal and professional identity act as one. As individuals become members of the profession, they are so identified with the profession that their membership in it cannot be separated from their personal identity. 'I am a nurse' is a statement that enumerates who I am, not just what I do" (p. 29). Nurses often work day, PM, and night shifts, but they are clearly on duty and accountable all day, every day.*

The Power of Others: Contributing to Change

In addition to nurses themselves, schools, health care and professional organizations, and the media are all in a position to strengthen the male nursing workforce. By promoting the profession of nursing to men, these leaders and organizations will help change a culture that has been slow to accept men.

Schools

Schools can lay the foundation for a less gendered view of nursing. Just as the power of one nurse can profoundly impact people's view of the profession, so can one teacher, guidance counselor, recruiter, or administrator. Staff in these and other leadership roles can educate and direct students to learn more about the nursing profession. These leaders need to have an understanding of the nursing profession and of the educational requirements and options for nursing education. With a basic knowledge about nursing and an enthusiasm for encouraging and directing students to explore educational and career options, teachers, guidance counselors, recruiters, and administrators can guide and influence students considering nursing as a profession.

Schools districts (especially high schools) can offer a curriculum designed to improve diversity, to expose students to health care careers and professionals, and to emphasize health care service standards like teamwork, leadership, compassion, and initiative. Many school districts already have this type of curriculum, called their *Health Academy*. In the Health Academy model, the school district partners with local health care organizations and liberal arts and technical colleges to develop curriculum and learning opportunities designed to provide students with health care-related college preparatory instruction. Classes, field-based learning, and the opportunity for students to have focused and consistent interactions with medical mentors are all designed to provide students with learning opportunities about health-related majors and careers.

Common Health Academy programs include classes, projects, and hands-on learning opportunities in areas such as anatomy and physiology, medical terminology, patient confidentiality (Health Insurance Portability and Accountability

Act [HIPAA]), cardiopulmonary resuscitation, nurse aide training, and in some cases, language arts courses with specific health care applications. Young men who participate in programs like the Health Academy not only learn about nursing, but they also can choose a male nurse for their medical mentor and observe male nursing role models and leaders. Programs like the Health Academy can greatly influence young people's view of our profession.

Colleges

Colleges with schools of nursing can promote the concept of gender diversity in a number of ways, including the following:

- In their strategic plan

- With their admissions committee

- In marketing and recruiting materials

- By hiring high-quality male faculty members

- With student nurse advisors

Teachers, guidance counselors, recruiters, and administrators at junior colleges and colleges without schools of nursing can also work to acquire a basic understanding of the educational requirements and options for nursing education.

General Organizations

Attracting men to the nursing profession has always been challenging, but health care organizations can encourage men to join the nursing workforce in a variety of ways. First, all organizations have strategic plans. These plans likely include language related to attracting and retaining nursing staff. Just as the American Nurses Credentialing Center's Magnet Recognition Program recognizes organizations for "quality patient care, nursing excellence and innovations in professional nursing practice" (American Nurses Credentialing Center [ANCC],

2012), it also lists attracting and retaining top talent and fostering a collaborative culture among the benefits of Magnet designation. The premise behind Magnet recognition is that organizations are recognized for attracting and retaining nurses.

Although these strategic plans are probably gender neutral, they should incorporate some of the IOM *Future of Nursing* report's aims. Just as the *Future of Nursing* aim 2 addresses the need for gender diversity in the nursing workforce (IOM, 2010a), so, too, should each organization include the need for gender diversity in its strategic plan. Inclusion of this language in an organization's strategic plan acknowledges a commitment to a goal or principle that is important to an organization's mission, its employees, and the populations they serve.

Organizations committed to increasing the number of men in their nursing workforce need to begin by attracting men to their organization as a whole. Successful organizations strive to be great places to work, and great workplaces begin by attracting a diverse group of quality employees.

One of the simplest, and perhaps most effective, strategies for attracting and recruiting employees is to shape an organization's reputation as a great place to work. Reputations, like culture, evolve over long periods of time. Satisfied employees tell others, thus building and cementing the organization's reputation. Organizations that have fostered a workplace culture that is supportive of men in nursing have achieved one of the most important goals for attracting male nurses. In addition to establishing a reputation as a great place to work, an organization can take specific steps and strategies to attract male nurses. Nurse recruiters, administrators, and the departments of human resources and marketing are among the key positions and departments for attracting men to an organization.

Nurse Recruiters

Nurse recruiters hold a key position to attract more men to the nursing workforce. A skilled nurse recruiter is also sensitive to the gender-specific needs of male and female nurses. The nurse recruiter works closely with an organization's department of human resources and nursing leaders to attract quality candidates to their organization. These nurse recruiters attend job and career fairs, participate in planning corporate advertising, and work with nurse managers and candidates to find positions that match a candidate's skills and needs. A nurse recruiter who is sensitive to the gender disparity in nursing and who works hard to meet the unique needs of all candidates can strengthen the male nursing workforce.

Nurse Managers

Nurse managers (head nurse, unit manager, chief nursing officer, and so on) are instrumental in creating a unit, department, or organization's culture. By listening to, responding to, and valuing the needs of their nurses, these nurse leaders create a culture that not only accepts but also promotes diversity in nursing.

Marketing Departments

A marketing department is an important part of an organization's plan to attract men to their nursing staff. A marketing department that is sensitive to and recognizes the need for gender diversity and works to communicate this value to its customers is important to an organization that is committed to a strong male presence among its nurses. Marketing department staff can work closely with the nursing department to include images and testimonials of men in their recruitment materials recognize the need for male nurses to work with recruitment staff as they participate in career fairs, and recognize the contributions of men in organizational newsletters and the local media.

Health Care Organizations

Health care organizations such as hospitals, nursing homes, and health departments can show their commitment to strengthening

the male nursing workforce in a number of ways, including the
following:

- By appointing men to key organizational work
  groups and committees

- By recognizing male nurse leaders and promoting
  them to leadership positions

- By implementing employee health and fitness and
  wellness activities that are gender neutral and
  appealing to men

- By designing or utilizing nurse satisfaction surveys
  that are gender neutral

- By using employee recognition tools and events that
  are appealing to men

Organizations such as the ANA, state/local/student nursing
organizations, and national organizations such as the National
Institutes of Health and the Robert Wood Johnson Foundation
are just a few of many that support nursing and health care.
These organizations have been instrumental in supporting
nursing. They have embraced opportunities to attract more
men to nursing by using gender-neutral terms in their policies
and education materials, by including images of men on their
websites and in their advertising by including male nurses in key
organizational positions, by publishing articles that support the
male nursing workforce, and by supporting research designed to
explore and understand the gender disparity in nursing.

> **NOTE**
>
> *As mentioned earlier, the AAMN, through its strategic
> plan, objectives, programs, and staff, is devoted to sup-
> porting men in nursing. This prominent national organiza-
> tion has chapters, leaders, and members throughout the
> country, and is a leader in planning and implementing
> strategies to attract men to the profession. They also have
> a useful resources page at http://aamn.org/resources.shtml.*

Nurse Researchers, Leaders, and Administrators

Collectively, nurse researchers, leaders, and administrators compose the final group that can strengthen the male nursing workforce. Nurse researchers have studied issues pertaining to men in nursing for decades. They have been, and will continue to be, instrumental in helping us learn what men consider as they contemplate nursing as a career choice. Nurse researchers also help us understand issues such as gender-based stereotypes, attitudes, barriers to recruitment, retention, nurse satisfaction, and many more issues that directly affect men in nursing.

Once the issues that contribute to the small male nursing workforce are identified, nurse leaders and change experts can plan, initiate, and evaluate improvement projects. Formal project improvement plans, such as plan, do, study, act (PDSA) projects, can be implemented.

The Role of the Media

Through printed material, radio, television, and movies, the media have limitless opportunities to display positive images of nursing—especially of men in nursing. Unfortunately, negative, inaccurate, sensationalized, or humorous images of nursing, and especially men in nursing, are more the norm. The media's timely, sensitive, and positive portrayals of men in nursing will play a key part in breaking stereotypes and promoting positive images of men in nursing. More advertisements with strong images of male nurses, captions like "Are You Man Enough to Be a Nurse" (2002) or "Iron Sharpens Iron" (AAMN, n.d.) and strong characters like the nurse "John" (portrayed by rock star Lenny Kravitz) in the Academy Award-nominated film *Precious* are needed to expose the public and men of all ages to nursing as a rewarding and socially acceptable profession for men.

Opportunities to strengthen the male nursing workforce are innumerable, but all involved must understand the change won't happen overnight. Perhaps the key can be found in yet another history lesson from the Roman Empire: "Rome wasn't built in a day." But using the Vitruvian concepts of durability, usefulness, and beauty, over time we can build a robust male nursing workforce to last.

MEN IN NURSING SURVIVAL TIPS: STRENGTHENING THE MALE NURSING WORKFORCE

First, any plan to strengthen the male nursing workforce must be consistent with the Vitruvian concepts of durability, usefulness, and beauty.

Second, changes to strengthen the male nursing workforce depend on an evidence-based process. Utilizing a model like Kotter's process for leading change will give nurse leaders and project planners a framework to guide them.

Third, every nurse (whether man or woman) has opportunities to strengthen the male nursing workforce. As a role model in the workplace, in the community, and as an outspoken advocate for nursing, every nurse can promote nursing as a great profession for men.

Fourth, health care employers, organizations like the ANA and AAMN, schools, nurse researchers and leaders, and the media must be engaged in this change. Their sensitivity, attention, and dedication to the roles they play in strengthening the male nursing workforce will be an important part of any plan.

The fifth and perhaps most important point is that strengthening the male nursing workforce will take time and the effort of many people, groups, and organizations.

References

American Assembly for Men in Nursing (AAMN). (n.d.). Iron sharpens iron. Retrieved from http://aamn.org/img/ad.Iron.h.1.jpg

American Assembly for Men in Nursing (AAMN). (2011). About us. Retrieved from http://aamn.org/aamn.shtml

American Assembly for Men in Nursing (AAMN). (2013). Strategic plan. Retrieved from http://aamn.org/docs/2013_strategic_plan.pdf

American Association of Colleges of Nursing (AACN). (2012). Retireved from http://www.aacn.nche.edu/research–data/standard–data–reports

American Nurses Association (ANA). (2012). *Code of ethics for nurses.* Retrieved from http://www.nursingworld.org/MainMenuCategories/EthicsStandards/CodeofEthicsforNurses

American Nurses Credentialing Center (ANCC). (2012). Program overview. Retrieved from http://www.nursecredentialing.org/Magnet/ProgramOverview

Are you man enough to be a nurse? [poster]. (2002). Retrieved from http://www.oregoncenterfornursing.org/index.php?mode=postersandmore

Institute of Medicine (IOM). (2010a). Report brief. *The future of nursing: Leading change, advancing health.* Retrieved from http://www.iom.edu/~/media/Files/Report%20Files/2010/The-Future-of-Nursing/Future%20of%20Nursing%202010%20Report%20Brief.pdf

Institute of Medicine (IOM). (2010b). *The future of nursing: Leading change, advancing health report recommendations.* Retrieved from http://www.iom.edu/~/media/Files/Report%20Files/2010/The-Future-of-Nursing/Future%20of%20Nursing%202010%20Recommendations.pdf

Kotter, J. P. (1996). *Leading change.* Boston, MA: Harvard Business School Press.

Porter-O'Grady, T. & Malloch, K. (2013). *Leadership in nursing practice: Changing the landscape of health care.* Burlington, MA: Jones & Bartlett Learning

Chapter 8
Leadership: A Matter of "Refereed" Experience

Franklin Shaffer, EdD, RN, FAAN
CEO, CGFNS International

When we look for good art, we look for a "juried" art show, where a panel of experts chooses only the best art works. When we need access to the most valid research, we look in "refereed" journals only. All this is well and good, but despite the plethora of literature on the subject of leadership, reading the literature will not help you become a leader. Leadership skills can be acquired a number of ways—through mentorships, training programs, on the job experience, and so forth. However, they are not acquired by reading a book! The reason for this is that leadership skills are primarily learned, tried, and tested through experience (Zelinsky, 1991).

Whether they are male or female, many nursing leaders believe that all leaders need the same characteristics; that people excel owing to these characteristics; and that neither intelligence nor "caring" are gender specific. The differences in how individual nurses actualize the nursing role account for varying levels of success. Indeed, this might be so, but gender plays a significant part in who you are and how you actualize your potential. If gender bias exists as an unrecognized, unaddressed component of nursing education programs, the outcomes degrade the profession and limit our ability to recruit and retain a robust workforce (Anthony, 2006).

Most male nurses want to be seen as nurses, not as "male nurses." They want to be part of the whole, not a highly visible minority (Davidson, 1996). Traditionally, men choose nursing for a variety of reasons that, in years past, differed from women's reasons:

- The desire to work in a humanistic field

- Nursing's emphasis on the biological sciences

- An opportunity to work in an administrative role

- Perhaps because, for one reason or another, they were unable to attend medical school

(Meadus & Twomey, 2007)

Today, however, both male and female nurses are likely to share a similar mix of reasons for choosing their profession (Boughn, 2001).

Are There Leadership Gender Differences?

Although the various dimensions of leadership are the same for both men and women (see Table 8.1 later in the chapter), very real differences exist in how men and women actualize these dimensions. For example, "A few [of these] characteristics particularly distinguish women from their male counterparts in the workplace. First, women can more often opt out of it [leadership] than men can. Second, their double burden—motherhood and management—drains energy in a particularly challenging way. Third, they tend to experience emotional ups and downs more often and more intensely than most men do"

(Barsh, Cranston, & Craske, 2008, para. 7). With regard to unpopular decisions, another female leader noted, "...[Male] General Managers say 'stop whining—man up, suck it up and shut up.' A female approach was completely different. I recognized that in order for this change to work, there had to be a quid pro quo" (Spencer, 2011, para. 6). In 1990, Eagly and Johnson published a meta-analysis of research on gender-related differences in leadership styles. Despite commonly held beliefs that women are more sensitive to the interpersonal dimensions of leadership and that men are more inclined to be task-oriented, the authors found no evidence of such differences among persons in leadership roles. However, among informal leaders (those not selected for a specific leadership role) the researchers found that women tended to adopt democratic leadership styles, whereas men tended to adopt an autocratic leadership style (Eagly & Johnson, 1990). This fascinating and unexpected finding seems to indicate that avoiding gender stereotypes may be the key to successful promotion to the formal leadership ranks.

However, in *Management and Leadership for Nurse Administrators,* Roussel, Swansburg, and Swansburg (2006) refer to Rosener's 1990 work "Ways Women Lead" and note that Rosener seems to think that men and women do operate differently when they are in leadership positions: "Rosener's work...indicates men operate more often through management transactions, exchanging rewards for services rendered or punishments for poor performance. Men also work more out of the power of their positions" (Roussel et al., 2006, p. 174).

These sources indicate gender does influence leadership styles and competencies. The quote from Roussel et al. (2006) notes that masculinity often results in task-oriented leaders who use direct approaches in decision-making. Femininity seems to allow a more people/person-oriented leadership approach, perhaps because women usually feel comfortable relating one-on-one with people at all levels of an organization. Businesswomen make it a point to be inclusive and to know the names and faces of the people with whom they work. Businessmen, however, tend to be more impersonal and usually do not interact with people at all levels of the organization.

Men tend to be more exclusive than inclusive. For women the term *inclusive* carries with it an implicit acknowledgement that people come first, whereas men place a higher value on objectivity, autonomy, and justice (Roussel et al., 2006). Eagly and Johnson indicate that there are minor stereotypic gender differences in some areas of leadership—women were more interpersonally oriented and more democratic, but none in other areas—for example, there were no sex differences among task comparisons. "Yet the mean effect size for interpersonal style was quite small. The largest overall sex difference was obtained for the democratic versus autocratic comparisons" (Eagly & Johnson 1990).

It is fair to conclude that leadership style, although gender-influenced, is not gender-specific, and for your own success you want to understand the differences and remain flexible enough to adapt your style to the situation. Leadership styles do not necessarily translate into good or bad; rather different styles may be more effective in some circumstances than in others. Therefore, you want to remain flexible enough to adapt your style to the situation.

What Makes a Successful Leader?

At its core, leadership itself refers to the capacity to release and engage human potential in the pursuit of common cause. However, "academic leaders exercise their leadership within settings that have markedly different institutional purposes, cultures, and expectations than the organizations in which business leaders typically exercise their leadership" (Moore & Diamond, 2000). As you consider a career in nursing leadership your ability to positively influence your peers and colleagues is a necessary ingredient for success. At this juncture, you are probably wondering, "What traits do I need?" Or, you might be thinking, "How can I succeed in a female-dominated profession?" Here are some pearls of wisdom I have learned from male colleagues in nursing leadership.

- **First, know your context.** It is essential to have a sense of clarity about your work environment. For some, this can be challenging, particularly when transitioning from clinical to the academic world. In the clinical world, you are advancing the mission of your practice setting, and in the academic world, you advance the blueprint of the university. So in essence, you need to read the mission statement of your workplace to understand the context of your leadership.

- **Second, do your homework.** This will require you to research the history of the organization and gain a sense of what worked and what caused stagnation. My colleagues told me this is the easiest misstep for a new leader when entering into a new workplace.

- **Third, surround yourself with those who are not afraid to disagree with your point of view.** Leaders must be willing to hear ideas that at times are in direct conflict with their own.

- **Fourth, be willing to revisit an issue that others deemed closed.** Sometimes a fresh look at an old problem can yield new solutions.

Finally, as a male nurse leader, you will bring a unique perspective for how to execute leadership from your life experience, and that is okay. However, I strongly encourage you to know your context, do your homework, be open to opposing perspectives, and be willing to revisit closed issues as you pursue this path.

Whereas leadership per se might not be situational, the styles and techniques used by leaders vary according to the situation. Bennis and Nanus suggest that you can find little consistency in the surface features of successful leaders: "They were right-brained, left-brained, tall and short, fat and thin, articulate and inarticulate, assertive and retiring, dressed for success and dressed for failure, participative and autocratic. Even their managerial styles were restlessly unruly" (Bennis & Nanus, 1985). What makes for a successful leader in an academic setting differs from what makes a leader successful in a business setting. In general, leaders in hospitals and other businesses tend toward transactional leadership styles, whereas leaders in education and educational institutions tend toward more transformative styles of leadership. However some men combine both styles and, in doing so, they become outstanding in both arenas.

CASE STUDY: LUTHER CHRISTMAN, NURSING'S MAN FOR ALL SEASONS

No one could discuss nursing, leadership, and men in nursing without acknowledging the trailblazing contributions of Luther Christman. A coal miner's son, he began his studies in 1936 as a student in the school for men at the Institute of Pennsylvania, but the Depression forced him to find a school that provided room, board and a small stipend. Dorothy Black, his high school sweetheart from Summit Hill, Pennsylvania, chose the Methodist Hospital School of Nursing in Philadelphia, and he soon followed. They married after finishing their studies for nursing. He experienced a great deal of gender discrimination as a man in a woman's profession in a less progressive time. "He was called a pervert when requesting maternity experience. He was refused admission to the Army Nurse Corps in World War II and entry to two university nursing programs simply because he was a man. Undeterred, Christman gained qualifications in psychology and his research led to high-level appointments in university nursing facilities" (Pittman, 2006, back cover). He taught nursing in Camden, New Jersey, while studying at Temple University and completed his doctoral studies at Michigan State University in 1965. In 1967, he became the first male to become dean of a school of nursing— Vanderbilt University (Rush University Alumni, n.d.).

I have always believed that leadership qualities can transfer from one setting (a college or university) to another (a hospital or medical center). Luther Christman is a case in point. In 1972, he left Vanderbilt and went to Rush University College of Nursing in Chicago where he served not only as dean but also as vice president for nursing at Rush University Medical Center. It was there that he developed what came to be known as the "Rush Model," which integrated nursing practice and education and served as a model for nursing education worldwide. Upon establishing a doctorate in nursing program at the Rush University Medical Center, Christman was able to motivate nurses to pursue higher education. Widely known, respected and controversial, he was a member of the Institute of Medicine, National Academies of Science, a recipient of the American Nurses Association Jessie M. Scott Award and inductee in their Hall of Fame. He was awarded three honorary degrees and was among the first to become a Fellow of the American Academy of Nursing (Hut, 2011).

However, Christman never forgot the issue of equality for men in nursing—and for other minorities. At Vanderbilt, he was the first dean to hire African-American women as faculty members. He frequently spoke to the discrimination that he and other men faced in nursing and actively encouraged men to pursue nursing as a career. "While Dean and Director of Nursing at Vanderbilt, Christman ran for the presidency of the American Nurses Association at the 1968 Dallas, TX, meeting. His defeat in that election brought with it a sense of unfairness towards men in nursing, an issue he fought for the rest of his long professional career" (Halloran, 2011). In 1974, he helped

continues

found the National Male Nurse Association which was re-named the American Assembly for Men in Nursing, and he served as its chairman until his death in 2011.

In 1995, The American Academy of Nursing awarded Luther Christman its highest honor: he was declared a Living Legend in Nursing. He remained active into his 90s, reviewing books, speaking, and teaching—and to the end, mentoring and encouraging men to enter the profession.

Table 8.1 contrasts transactional and Transformative leadership. Initial studies portrayed transactional leadership and transformational leadership as mutually exclusive, but Bass and Bass, among others, view transactional and transformational leadership as a continuum rather than as opposites (Bass & Bass, 2008). The transformational leadership style complements the transactional style and will likely prove ineffective in the total absence of a transactional relationship between leaders and subordinates. To display the differences in a simple and effective manner, I have summarized the differences in Table 8.1.

TABLE 8.1 Transactional Versus Transformative Leadership

TRANSACTIONAL LEADERSHIP	TRANSFORMATIVE LEADERSHIP
Leaders are aware of the link between the effort and reward.	Leaders arouse emotions in their followers that motivate them to act beyond the framework of what may be described as exchange relations.
Leadership is responsive, and its basic orientation is dealing with present issues.	Leadership is proactive and forms new expectations in followers.
Leaders rely on standard forms of inducement, reward, punishment, and sanction to control followers.	Leaders create learning opportunities for their followers and stimulate followers to solve problems.

TRANSACTIONAL LEADERSHIP	TRANSFORMATIVE LEADERSHIP
Leaders motivate followers by setting goals and promising rewards for desired performance.	Leaders are distinguished by their capacity to inspire and provide individualized consideration, intellectual stimulation, and idealized influence to their followers.
Leadership depends on the leader's power to reinforce subordinates for their successful completion of the bargain.	Leaders possess good visioning, rhetorical, and management skills, the better with which to develop strong emotional bonds with followers.
	Leaders motivate followers to work for goals that go beyond self-interest.

According to Goleman, Boyatzis, and McKee, common leadership styles found in hospitals blend command, transactional, and bureaucratic styles. Bureaucratic leadership refers to "by the book" leadership—that is, the leader focuses on policy and procedures and seeks to keep things fair and well-organized. The commanding leader provides clear direction and makes all decisions. The two most common, but least effective, leadership styles they noted were pacesetting, where leaders establish challenge goals and enact those competitively, and the autocratic style, which is frequently misused and overused, and also minimally effective except in a crisis situation (Goleman, Boyatzis, & McKee, 2009). However, in contrast, two of the most effective styles are visionary (leaders direct and involve people by creating and communicating a particular vision) and coaching (leaders work with employees on developing and meeting long-term goals) (Goleman et al., 2009).

Hints for Successful Leadership

Many an unkind word has been said about *prima donnas*, but the term itself is a compliment: it means first, the best, the most acclaimed. Marks of respect for contributions made are not

"coddling" individuals, but rather appreciating achievement—
and holding it up for others to emulate.

Meetings are to be minimized as much as possible, but if
you must have meetings they should be both short and effective.
Never deceive others about the nature of the meeting. If
administration has adopted a decision, do not pretend the group
is free to come up with its own proposal.

HAVING SUCCESSFUL MEETINGS

*No meeting can be successful if you have not first clarified
the purposes of the get-together. You need to know—and
so do your team members—in advance which of the
following goals you are trying to accomplish:*

- *To give people essential information and to
  allow them to ask questions.*

- *To win support for a decision already made and
  to persuade the group to pitch in and make it a
  success.*

- *To present an unsolved problem to the group
  and elicit their thinking about how it can
  be handled. (You may want to take their
  recommendations under advisement or allow the
  group to make the actual decision. The objective
  should be clear in your own mind before you call
  the meeting to order.)*

If you agree with the policy or decision, you face little
difficulty. If you happen to be in disagreement, you have a
dilemma: to remain silent about your personal view or to
indicate your dissatisfaction. There are circumstances which can
justify either approach, but whatever decision you reach should
be based on a careful consideration of the consequences. Never
put yourself in a position where it can be said that you have

sabotaged a decision made by those in authority, that is, those who have been vested with the right to make the decision. Still, your own conscience or sense of personal dignity might compel you to indicate your own personal views. In that case, you are duty bound to make it clear that, despite your disagreement, you intend to carry out the institution's policy and to make it as workable as possible. The only other alternative would be to resign.

DEADLINES AND MILESTONES

Most people, no matter how good their sense of timing, find they need the discipline of deadlines to get things done. The practice of setting up milestones along the road into the future is constructive. However, deadlining must be intelligently implemented. If it is to be effective you must meet these conditions:

- *You must have a sense of how much time specific tasks require. Unless you have timed your own past performances, you may miss the boat in making new commitments. (Some of us have a tendency to overestimate, others to underestimate, how long a job will take. Examine your own record to find out in which group you belong, and make proper allowances in the future.)*

- *Fix sub-deadlines so that you can pace your activities to meet the overall deadline. This will allow you to check on whether you are really on schedule, ahead of schedule, or falling behind. In the latter case, you will know that you had better put on an extra spurt of energy.*

- *Include in your scheduling some time for anticipated interruptions, or if they cannot be anticipated, for unexpected events.*

If You Want to Succeed

Men like Lee Iacocca were leaders because they loved their work, which led to a passion for excellence, which in turn led them to teach other like-minded people. A shared passion creates cohesion. Iacocca didn't seek power for its own sake: in fact, he didn't seek it at all. His passion was his power. He didn't have to motivate others; his performance motivated them (we call this role modeling). He didn't try to develop them; correcting and encouraging are natural components of teaching (we call this coaching). Because he was good—and he knew it—he wasn't threatened by other leaders. He wasn't interested in the pecking order, and he already made enough money; watching youngsters excel is what gave him pleasure. And they loved him for it, and mourned when it when it was time for him to move onward and upward.

Success demands effective leadership. And effective leadership demands commitment to the work, the organization, and the position. Lack of leadership and lack of consistency leads to lack of follow through, and all three—changing positions, losing consistency, and failing to follow through—lead to loss of momentum. Moreover, successful enterprises run on an absolute minimum of meetings, but the meetings that they do have are worth their time. The most successful sport teams have members who belong to only one team at a time. Thus each team member focuses solely on this team's goal—and they are members by choice, their own and the team leader's. Moreover, they must be good at what they do to be chosen to be a member of the team. They are expected to be experts in their own fields and to respect the expertise of others. They are not expected to be their own marketers, accountants, purchasers, and managers. They have very specific assignments. Big name teams have big name stars. They allow people to stand out so long as they don't become arrogant and self-serving.

CASE STUDY: GENERAL WILLIAM BESTER—AN EXEMPLAR OF EXCELLENCE

William Bester started nursing school with an interest in becoming a nurse anesthetist. When he met a recruiter at the College of St. Scholastica, he entered a program called the Army Student Nurse Corps Program that paid tuition, books, and a stipend. This helped him get his BSN from the College of St. Scholastica in Duluth, Minnesota. After that he started serving his 3 years as an officer in the U.S. Army Nurse Corps. He graduated from the U.S. Army Nurse Anesthesia Program in Tacoma, Washington, in 1979. In 1985, he earned an MSN from Catholic University of America in Washington, DC.

In the academic world, Bester was best known for his prowess as a nurse leader. He served as a nurse anesthetist at Fort Chaffee, Arkansas (1980), and commanded a Medical Task Force as well as served in a major leadership role at Moncrief Army Community Hospital, Fort Jackson, South Carolina. In recognition of his leadership skills, the United States Army named Bester chief nursing officer. This recognition exemplified his commitment to excellence as well as his ability to recognize other nurses with exemplary clinical performance.

At a pivotal point in his career, Bester sought an academic role in a clinical setting at the University of Texas in Austin and an administrative leadership role at the Seton Family of Hospitals in Austin, Texas.

Bester, now a retired Brigadier General, oversees the External Affairs Division at the Uniformed Services University (USU). Prior to assuming this massive responsibility, Bester served as the Vice President and Acting Dean of the Graduate School of Nursing at USU. Subsequently, he served in a variety of leadership roles. He

continues

is a sought-out speaker because of his expertise in nursing leadership and management of disasters. The American Assembly for Men in Nursing (AAMN) awarded Bester the coveted Luther Christman Reward. Additionally, he was granted an honorary doctorate from two universities. Bester was also recognized for distinguished military service as the recipient of notable military medals. Finally, he holds active memberships in major nursing associations such as Sigma Theta Tau International. Bester's career exemplifies the impact male nurse leaders can have who develop a prudent blueprint for success. His career is the personification of leadership and should inspire you to follow the pearls of wisdom previously described in this chapter: to know your context, do your homework, surround yourself with those who are willing to disagree with your point of view, and be willing to revisit an issue considered closed.

The Case for Ethical Leadership

Like all their administrative predecessors and models, health leaders derive their political and social advantages from their power to allocate the limited resources assigned to their discretion. Moreover, chief nursing officers derive their moral authority to allocate resources from their clinical knowledge and professional commitments, under the expectation that these moderate the contractual (self-interest) model of marketplace behavior. As both nurses and leaders, executive nurses are concerned about both nursing ethics and business ethics. Although these two are not inimical, they derive from different traditions that, in some cases, may lead to different conclusions (Brown, 2006).

The fallout from the recent corporate scandals—scandals affecting nearly every industry in America, from Enron and

Arthur Andersen to Tenet and the Sisters of Mercy Health System—has made it abundantly clear that the business ethos in our country is woefully inadequate to contemporary ethical challenges. Meticulously high standards of conduct are crucial to the welfare of the corporation, its people, and to all affected by its operations. We have all seen the high costs that corporate scandals have exacted: heavy fines, jail time for corporate leaders, destruction of security and retirement funds, investors defrauded of life savings, a 1,000% increase in serious errors in U.S. hospitals, low morale, recruiting difficulties, internal fraud, and loss of public confidence (Ciulla, 2004).

Therefore, you must adopt a covenantal ethic (an ethic that suggests that all parties in such a commercial endeavor should benefit on the basis of created value and the voluntary exchange of resources) that more fully addresses the problems unique to providing essential human services within a competitive marketplace (Nash, 1990). Whereas the contractual model focuses on profit as the first purpose and other-oriented values as a secondary contractual condition, the covenantal approach has as its first purpose the welfare of others and views profit as a secondary contractual condition. Whereas the customary contractual model of business ethics regards efficiency measures as a primary focus of problem solving and benefit to others (greatest good for the greatest number) as an assumed result, the covenantal ethic sees the creation of mutually enabling relationships as the assumed result, and it sees servicing relationships as the primary vehicle for problem solving (Curtin, 2011).

Under this covenant, return on investment (ROI) is acknowledged as an essential component of business, but the receipt of a legitimate return is absolutely conditional on the creation and provision of value in other people's terms. Thus, ROI is transformed from being a primary purpose to a secondary result—that is, financial results are the byproducts of other measures of performance. From an ethical perspective, the covenantal ethic draws on very different values to guide and mold decision-making. A commitment to service rather than to a single-minded pursuit of corporate self-interest is the spark that ignites problem solving. By fixating on this commitment, leadership begins to see business as a series of enabling relationships rather than as a set of efficiency measures.

The effect of this change in purpose on managerial problem definition is profound. Instead of asking, "Is our market share growing? How can I arrange my resources to grow?" a manager asks, "What does the community need? How can I gather the resources to provide it?" Instead of chaining your outlook to milking the status quo, you try to build on it. Service and value creation become intrinsically important *on their own*. As a building block of quality, such assumptions are a far stronger appeal, particularly to health professionals, than an appeal to profit (Nash, 1990).

CASE STUDY: DAVID BENTON—A STRONG AND GRACIOUS GLOBAL LEADER

David Benton took the position as chief executive officer of the International Council of Nurses (ICN) on 1 October 2008. Immediately prior to this he worked with ICN for 3 years where he held the role of consultant for nursing and health policy and specialized in regulation, licensing, and education. He is currently completing his PhD in Nursing. I have the good fortune of knowing David Benton as a friend and a colleague. He made me feel very welcomed when I attended the ICN in Malta where I was first introduced to the world of nursing as the CEO of CGFNS International. I have learned much from him. He is the type of person who has a genuine interest in others and a passion for nursing. He maximizes his position to advocate for nurses in the World Health Organization, the Organization for Economic Cooperation and Development, USAID, World Bank, and other international business and social organizations. His is a strong, multilingual voice for nursing—and for men in nursing.

During his graduate studies Benton focused on how computers could improve nursing education. This led to several influential publications that influenced the practice of nursing education. Throughout his career he served in multiple leadership roles within the health care system.

He is well traveled both nationally and internationally. During his travels he extensively examined the health systems of the United States and other countries that facilitated his capacity to carve out a voice for nurses within the Scottish health system. Benton has been recognized with many accolades including the inaugural Nursing Standard Leadership award in 1993. Additionally, he was elected to a Fellowship of the Florence Nightingale Foundation in 2001 and the Royal College of Nursing in 2003 for his numerous outstanding contributions to the profession. Benton's career is another exemplar of how male nurse leaders have prominently transformed the role of male nurses. Similar to Bester, he forged a path of excellence by increasing his knowledge about the context of the different health care systems, and by doing the necessary homework about these systems, he developed strategies and allies that earned him esteemed recognition by the nursing profession.

Recognizing that the ethical challenges of today's health care system cannot be glossed over with public relations expertise, yet another congressional hearing, or even the development of new and comprehensive quality standards, Nash, in particular, offers a well-grounded, but workable approach to developing leaders who can deal practically with the moral problems inherent in the daily operations of a health services corporation. By focusing on real-world dilemmas that emphasize the relationship between good ethics and good business and using examples drawn from extensive experience, Nash describes situations where ethical assumptions and commercial decisions are inextricably connected. By offering a set of practical questions about decisions and actions (Could I disclose this to the public? Does this action pass the "stink test"? Am I hurting anyone?), Nash shows how leaders can get back in touch with the values that define the health professions—and the values that created a prosperous economy (Nash, 1990).

Ethical and effective leadership is likely to prove even more essential in the future to facilitate the growth and adaptation of human services organizations in the constant challenge to improve performance. This will require not only individual leadership development but also greater attention to teaching leadership in schools of social work and to others preparing human services managers. In the end, leadership has little to do with your gender. Rather it is the outcome of a passion for what you do, a whole-hearted commitment to excellence and both the intelligence and the stamina to stay the course.

MEN IN NURSING LEADERSHIP SURVIVAL TIPS

While it is necessary to seek a strong male mentor, it is also wise to seek a female leader to help mentor you.

Build an extensive network of professional colleagues of both genders.

Join the Assembly for Men in Nursing, and become active members of the American Nurses Association and also your specialty organization, for example, AORN, AACN, AONE, etc.

Seek to combine the best traits of transformative and transactional leadership.

References

Anthony, A. S. (2006). Tear down the barriers of gender bias. *Men in Nursing, 1*(4), 43-49.

Barsh, J., Cranston, S., & Craske, R. A. (2008). Centered leadership: How talented women thrive. *McKinsey Quarterly,* September 2008. Retrieved from http://www.mckinseyquarterly.com/ Centered_leadership_How_talented_women_thrive_2193

Bass, B., & Bass, R. (2008). *The Bass handbook of leadership: Theory, research, and managerial applications (4th ed.).* New York, NY: Free Press.

Bennis, W. G., & Nanus, B. (1985). *Leaders: The strategies for taking charge.* New York, NY: Harper & Row.

Boughn, S. (2001). Why women and men choose nursing. *Nursing and Health Care Perspectives, 22*(1), 14-20.

Brown, B. J. (2006). Integrity, ethics and trust. *Nursing Administration Quarterly, 30*(1), 1-2.

Ciulla, J. B. (Ed.). (2004). *Ethics: The heart of leadership.* New York, NY: Praeger Publishers.

Curtin, L. (2011). Quantum leadership: Succeeding in interesting times. *Nursing Leadership, 9*(1), 35-38.

Davidson, M. (1996). Not a male nurse, a real nurse. *Nursing Forum, 31*(4), 28.

Eagly, A. H., & Johnson, B. T. (1990). Gender and leadership style: A meta-analysis. *Psychological Bulletin, 108*(2), 233-256.

Goleman, D., Boyatzis, R., & McKee, A. (2009). Primal leadership. *Leadership Excellence, 26*(10), 9-10.

Halloran, E. J. (2011). Luther P. Christman, 1915–2011. Retrieved from www.aamn.org/docs/luther_christman_obit.pdf

Hut, Nick. (2011). Pioneering nurse Luther Christman dies at 96. Retrieved from http://news.nurse.com/article/20110610/ NATIONAL02/306100017/-1/frontpage

Meadus, R. J., & Twomey J. C. (2007). Men in nursing: Making the right choice. *The Canadian Nurse, 103*(2), 13-16.

Moore, M. R., & Diamond, M. A. (2000). *Academic leadership: Turning vision into reality.* Ernst and Young Foundation.

Nash, L. L. (1990). *Good intentions aside: A manager's guide to resolving ethical problems.* Boston, MA: Harvard Business Review Press.

Pittman, E. (2006). Luther Christman: A maverick nurse—A nursing legend. Victoria, BC, Canada: Trafford Publishing.

Rosener, J. B. (1990). Ways women lead. *Harvard Business Review, 68*(6), 119-125.

Roussel, L., Swansburg, R. C., and Swansburg, R. L. (2006). *Management and leadership for nurse administrators, 4th edition.* Burlington, MA: Jones and Bartlett Learning.

Rush University Alumni. (n.d.). Founding Dean Christman shaped the field of nursing. Retrieved from http://con.rushalumni.org/Christman

Spencer, S. (2011). Women lead differently than men, and that's a good thing for business. Reuters online edition. Retrieved from http://blogs.reuters.com/great-debate/2011/03/08/women-lead-differently-than-men-and-thats-a-good-thing-for-business/

Zelinski, M. (1991). Outward bound: The inward odyssey. Hillsboro, OR: Beyond Words Publishing.

Chapter 9

Men in Academia: Pursuing a Career in Nursing Research

Joachim G. Voss, PhD, RN, ACRN
Associate Professor, University of Washington
Steven Simpkins, RN
PhD student, University of Washington
School of Nursing, Biobehavioral Nursing & Health Systems

Once you have better understood why a male might choose a female-dominated profession, have answered repeated questions about your sexual orientation (and left those stereotypes behind you), and have achieved expertise in your area of nursing practice, you stand at a crossroads in your career. This chapter covers a career plan in nursing research and offers a stepwise approach to pursuing a faculty position in academia. By intertwining personal experiences with scientific evidence, the chapter provides you a more complete picture of careers in nursing research.

Advanced Degrees

In the United States today, nursing education at the university level is divided into four categories:

- Bachelor's degree for entry into practice

- Master's degree or a docto in nursing practice (DNP) for delivery of advanced nursing practice

- Educational doctorate for becoming an expert teacher in nursing

- Doctor of philosophy (PhD), which focuses on achieving a role that combines academic research, education, and professional service activities

(Kim, McKenna, & Ketefian, 2006)

Nursing has lately made moves similar to other science fields such as medicine, pharmacy, social work, and physical therapy to have students enter directly from their bachelor of science in nursing (BSN) program into a research or clinical doctorate program (Nehls & Barber, 2011). Strong opinions inform this debate as to whether nurses should indeed be allowed to make such a transition before accumulating substantial clinical practice time. We favor the possibility of early entry into PhD programs in nursing and want to encourage more men to enter into a research career and thus have a longer and more productive career.

When nurses begin their PhD training later in life, they significantly shorten the time they have to establish themselves as successful researchers. This does not mean that they are not successful or productive, but their overall time in the research arena is limited to between 10 and 20 years as opposed to between 30 and 40 years. Men in nursing might not follow the same career pattern in nursing compared to women, as they usually do not take a family break. The men Joachim has have met in nursing always had stronger motivations for advancing their career earlier than women did and had a greater drive towards more leadership, more responsibilities, and greater financial independence. Despite these differences between the sexes, most applicants to U.S. doctoral programs select PhD training after they have been expert clinicians for a number of years (Harding, 2009). We believe, however, that only by recruiting and retaining younger men into nursing research can we fill the looming faculty gap resulting from the large numbers of retiring nurse faculty members over the next 5 years.

Experienced PhD applicants often have many advantages, though, because civilian and military health centers regularly participate in patient-focused research activities and do so with the help of BSN- and master's-prepared nursing staff. For many nurses, this offers an opportunity to develop an interest in and perhaps a passion for research. Nurses often decide to pursue a PhD after participation in randomized clinical trials, large cohort studies, or vaccine trials. They pique their curiosity, discover their own passion, develop their own research ideas, and realize that without proper training they are not fully prepared to lead their own research efforts (Jolley, 2007).

Major motivators for pursuing a career in research include the following:

- Drive for more independence
- Recognition of one's own creative potential
- Rewards of becoming a published and recognized scholar (Lou, Yu, & Chen, 2010)

This type of initial work experience provides insight into the need for scientific rigor, diligence, and patience required to become a successful researcher. Previous exposure to grant proposals, research protocols, study designs, and theoretical frameworks gives the potential applicant a better idea about the career that lies ahead (Nehls & Barber, 2011).

This chapter provides insight into critical questions for the preparation phase, covers a successful application process, discusses effective mentoring, describes various phases of the PhD program, develops a plan for pursuing a postdoctoral position, and presents a 5-year plan for the junior faculty phase.

Considering the Next Step

All potential PhD applicants must consider their stage of readiness for such a career move. This decision requires careful thought and staged planning. In the preparation phase, ask yourself the hard question of whether you can and want to leave a significant portion of your clinical practice behind to conduct independent research.

Although daily clinical practice takes its toll physically and emotionally, it is, at the same time, emotionally rewarding when patients and families master a crisis or overcome a serious illness. This is one reason why nurses find their profession so desirable and worthy of doing it for decades.

An important question to ask yourself is this: Am I ready to dedicate a significant portion of my work (at least 50%) toward writing manuscripts, proposals, recommendation letters, and reviews? Research work and dissemination of your results doesn't provide the instant gratification you receive from clinical work, and writing as a professional requirement for most nurses is unfamiliar, poses a significant challenge, and even seems threatening. In fact, you'll find that mentors, reviewers, classmates, and others will critique the content of your work repeatedly and sometimes harshly. Don't let harsh comments discourage you, though. Instead, see this as a challenge to improve your current product (Jolley, 2007).

Another question you need to answer: Can you accept leaving behind the comfort of your expert role and return to a novice status in nursing research? Most nurses decide to venture into the PhD program when they are mid-career, have established sound relationships, have formed a close social network, and have potentially started a family (Meachin & Webb, 1996; Nehls & Barber, 2011). To reestablish a life in a new environment all while facing the academic challenges that lie ahead, potential candidates often put off or give up these comforts and sometimes even physically move far away. This soul searching goes hand in hand with the decision of where to pursue your degree. Factors you want to consider include the following:

- What institution can you afford financially?

- How will you find a close mentor to guide you through the academic jungle?

- What financial offerings does the institution have to support you and your family?

(Kjellgren, Welin, & Danielson, 2005)

Other important activities have proven beneficial for a successful PhD transition, too, including the following:

- Previous engagement with specialty organizations

- Research engagement

- Leadership positions in nursing

- Engagement in health policy efforts

- Dissemination of your opinions in regional or national professional meetings

- Publication experience

(Marsland & Hickey, 2003)

> **NOTE**
>
> *If you feel uncertain about any of these factors, you might find entry into a PhD program more difficult, but not impossible with the guidance of a strong mentor.*

Leaving Your Clinical Practice

To leave a significant portion of clinical practice behind is the greatest challenge for many BSN, master's, and DNP students; however, they will find it very difficult to stay engaged with a demanding hospital position while transitioning into a nursing researcher role (Rodts & Lamb, 2008). Very few BSN graduates come to their PhD programs with a clinical research question that they develop while in the BSN program. In contrast, master's or DNP graduates often discover their passion and interest for a particular area of research through working as clinical nurse specialists or nurse practitioners. They then enter the PhD program with clear research questions and pursue those with great diligence.

All future researchers should answer at some point in their training how much they want to stay engaged with a particular clinical population. How might you stay engaged within your area of expertise? Well, you have a variety of options:

- You can continue to provide some direct care.

- You can serve on the board of a patient organization.

- You can join a professional nursing organization.

- You can become active in health policy in your specialty area.

These few examples show how you might stay engaged and current with your area of expertise. They are independent of your requirements for the PhD and can benefit your future faculty career. The ultimate goal of a nursing researcher should always be aimed at improvements for the population you want to serve: *your patients, your communities,* and *your country.*

KEEPING CURRENT

One example of continuous engagement that has worked for Joachim is being part of a professional organization. The Association of Nurses in AIDS Care helps him stay current on issues of prevention, diagnosis, and treatment in HIV care. He is part of the local chapter board, and it organizes an annual clinical conference for around 100 nurses on HIV-related care topics. He goes to the annual National Conference to share his research experiences, meet colleagues and discuss new ideas, and attend free seminars to keep my knowledge current. Activities such as this ensure engagement with clinical colleagues and familiarity with the most recent trends that you will someday want to share with your own students.

Academic Writing

Another consideration as you prepare to make your decision to pursue a PhD is scientific writing, an activity that every academic must undertake. Your progress through the academic ranks depends on it, honors and awards often come with it, and your scholarly reputation grows with it (Jolley, 2007). Most academics find writing a manuscript, a proposal, or any other document difficult and burdensome. It requires time, careful thought, and strict attention to detail in following written guidelines.

You can learn good scientific writing, though, so you should take as many academic writing workshops as you possibly can. By doing so, you will find your own voice and become a better writer. You will also learn the process and structure of how to provide constructive feedback for other writers (including your future students). Writing should become a daily activity so that it does not become a painful task that you shy away from (Jolley, 2007). What is really surprising for us is that in the last 10 years in nursing, 30% of all nursing-related publications have been published by male first authors. Again, this is an indicator to our previous point for men having strong career drives and the desire for more independence and recognition (Shields, Hall, & Mamun, 2011).

NOTE

Academic writing is important not only while you're pursuing a degree. All researchers have the responsibility to share their study findings with the larger research community. Only then does the research exist and truly enter the academic community for discussion and debate. Anything less and you just waste time and valuable resources.

Are You Really Ready?

Long before you begin the application process, you and your future mentor should evaluate the question of whether you are at a good stage in your life to make this critical decision.

CAUTION

An impending pregnancy, a severely sick partner or other family member, or your partner's loss of employment are just a few examples of where a good mentor might caution you against entering a PhD program.

As you embark on your academic career, your life needs to be emotionally and financially stable (Jolley, 2007). This means that you are not planning a marriage, going through a divorce, or participating in an adoption program. Carefully discuss all these details with your potential mentor to give the mentor the chance to guide you from personal experience. The fewer emotional and financial changes that might distract from your PhD, the greater is your chance of successfully completing your degree. Committing to a 4-year academic program is an emotional and financial burden not only for you but also for your partner, your family, and your friends (Rodts & Lamb, 2008).

Pre-Application Planning

In preparing for this formidable task, you must do some intensive research. Download the application requirements for all research-intensive schools under consideration. Make a table for yourself that lists the factors for choosing each institution, and includes the following:

- Location

- Reputation

- Cost

- Potential mentors in the area of your interest

- Funding programs and scholarships opportunities through the school or the university

- Requirements for completion of the PhD

- Number of annual PhD students who graduate

- Housing opportunities

   (Kjellgren et al., 2005)

Defining an area of interest prior to your application to a school will greatly increase your chances of identifying a good mentor/mentee fit. Finding the best personal connection is one way to ensure that you have the right person who will devote considerable amounts of time to your progression and success throughout the program (Nehls & Barber, 2011). This also proves a major advantage as you prepare to complete your application.

When you approach a potential mentor, always come with a standard set of questions that you use for every interview so that you can make comparisons. Factors to help you determine whether you have a good fit might include the following:

- Their most recent research projects

- How many mentees they currently have

- How often they usually meet with mentees

- Whether their students have received any scholarships

- Whether they teach in the PhD program

- Their involvement (or not) in the curriculum of the PhD program

- The average time to graduate for their students

- Whether their students have found postdoctoral or junior faculty positions

Make a table and rate the faculty you meet. Most likely, you will need at least three to five of these conversations to make a proper comparison and arrive at a sound decision. You can conduct these interviews with faculty members from within the same university or across different institutions.

> **NOTE**
>
> *One major guide in your assessment should be your own personal impression of whether you think this mentor and you are compatible for a 4-year or more commitment. If you do not like someone during your first meeting, that person is most likely not the best fit for you. Compatibility of personality has a major impact on your future success, and so you should consider it a major factor in your search for the most supportive and interesting candidate (Rodts & Lamb, 2008).*

Such conversations can happen formally at an institution or very informally at community meetings where the faculty member is a guest speaker. If you do not have the money to spend on travel, you can in many cases use Internet video connections that enable you to have face-to-face conversations with a potential mentor while avoiding the costs of travel (Kim et al., 2006). In preparation for these conversations, read their publications relevant to your interest, search their curriculum vitae (CV)/biography on the Internet, learn their affiliations in your area of interest, and come prepared and informed.

Now that personal connections have been established, your core questions shift to the requirements for the PhD application. Do I need to document a GRE score? If so, how do I study for and take the test? If I have already taken the test, how old is the score? Do I need to retake it? Foreign students must take an English proficiency test and achieve a certain score; in addition, they need a student visa for the United States. What about funding for your PhD program? While almost everyone finds funding difficult, it is especially so for foreign students. Finding scholarships through their government, the Fulbright Program, or other institutions can be a lengthy process and may require substantial amounts of time (see Table 9.1).

These types of administrative requirements demand enormous attention to detail and often take up to 12 months or more to complete, especially for international applicants. So, create a checklist with required due dates for the completion of these tasks to ensure that you do not forget important submission deadlines, particularly if you plan to send your application to different organizations (Williams & Jordan, 2007).

Being a man in nursing and competing against female colleagues can be difficult. You are often the only man among female colleagues. In the U.S. only a low percentage of nurses are men, and in academia the numbers are smaller. Competing for funding as a man in nursing does not get easier but harder.

If you apply to any nursing organization, your proposal for any funding needs to be flawless and exceptional, so you stand out from the beginning and no one can say later that you only got this scholarship or training program because you are a man. You need to convince the reviewers with your abilities, your intellect, and your excellent ideas. Make sure multiple people have read the proposal and provided input so that you have heard multiple perspectives before you send it out for review.

TABLE 9.1 Mentor and Funding Phases for an Academic Career

PHASE	MENTORSHIP	FUNDING OPPORTUNITIES
Pre-doctoral	BSN mentor Future PhD mentor Nursing leader in a clinical setting Research mentor	Applications to Fulbright Commission, national scholarships, defense scholarships, school funding, student loans, and private funding
PhD training	PhD mentor Dissertation chair Dissertation advisor Academic services	National Institutes of Health funding (T-32 stipends), National Research Service Aware (NRSA) funding, small and large foundation funding
Postdoctoral	Postdoctoral mentor Academic colleagues Institute of Translational Health Sciences (ITHS) mentorship	Small and large foundation funding, intramural pilot study funding, R-34 funding, co-investigator on larger grant
Junior faculty	Department chair Dean for research Faculty mentor Faculty colleagues	NIH K-Awards and R-series funding, large foundation funding (Oncology Nursing Society [ONS], other disease societies), Department of Defense (DOD), Health Resources and Services Administration (HRSA), Gates Foundation

> **TIP**
>
> *Most of your reviewers in nursing will be women, so make sure you write your proposal in a style that your female colleagues can relate to. Consider reading some of the major feminist theory publications, for example, the works of Susan Sontag.*

The Application Process

Most PhD programs have online submission systems and require you to follow strict instructions. Admission boards consider deviation from these instructions as an inability to follow written instructions, and as a result, your application loses important points in the evaluation process or might be rejected outright. Even if you do not understand the purpose of the instructions, follow them or call the school to have someone explain the unclear parts of the application, especially if you are applying from outside the United States.

> **NOTE**
>
> *Because so few men apply to nursing PhD programs, you might have a slight advantage. Most nursing schools welcome gender diversity and will make an effort to accept male applicants. Again, making sure you have a complete application will be 50% of your entrance ticket. However, remember that no school of nursing will give you admission to their PhD program just because you are a man.*

Your Curriculum Vitae

The application usually requires you to submit a curriculum vitae (CV), which you should already have on hand; keep this updated at all times. This allows you to track your professional growth, documents your achievements, and allows the reviewers to see how you present yourself professionally. Format and content vary from institution to institution, and you can usually find instructions on how to format a CV on the institution's website. Keep in mind this important distinction: A CV is a detailed description of your professional past with attention to detail, whereas a biography is a summary of your most significant accomplishments. Most academic institutions want you to be detail oriented and complete so that your entire development is visible (Rodts & Lamb, 2008). Even if you spent time as a volunteer in a remote region of the world, document it; these details actually make an application stronger. The nearby sidebars give sample outlines for a CV and a biography. The CV can be lengthy as long as you have something important to say (mine [Voss] is currently 25 pages long), but the short bio shouldn't exceed 4 pages.

OUTLINE FOR CV CATEGORIES (ORDER DEPENDS ON THE INSTITUTION)

1. Demographics
   a. Name
   b. Present Position
   c. Address

2. Licensure & Certificates

3. Education

4. Professional Positions

5. Research Experience
   a. Grant name
   b. Principal investigator
   c. Agency
   d. Type of grant
   e. Time worked on the grant
   f. Role on the grant
   g. Brief goal statement of the grant

6. Publications

7. Presentations

8. Posters

9. Honors

10. Professional Memberships

11. Professional Activities

12. Service Activities

13. Teaching Activities

OUTLINE FOR PROFESSIONAL BIOGRAPHY (ORDER DEPENDS ON THE INSTITUTION)

1. Name and Current Title

2. Education

3. Honors

4. Short Goal Statement

5. Publications

6. Research Experience

Essays

The essay section forms the second critically important part of the application. These answer questions about activities and coursework that has prepared you for entry into the PhD program as well as the professional and personal experiences that contribute to the decision-making process of pursuing a research doctorate. Other questions might ask what you hope to gain from the completion of the program and what your career goals are. Yes, before you even start the program, faculty members want to know whether you have thought about a trajectory for your future. As part of your admission to the PhD program of any School of Nursing (SON), faculty in those schools will welcome and see you as their future colleagues; so, it is in their best interest to fully understand your intentions and to provide you with the personal and educational resources to take on this new role and fulfill their expectations.

An important part of the essays deals with your research interest. This refers to a particular area of nursing that you think is critically underdeveloped. BSN-prepared applicants have a clear disadvantage here because they were often not as involved in clinical research and, therefore, have less of a focus entering a PhD program. So this means getting engaged in research during your undergraduate education is of great value. Talk to your peers and to your professors about how you might go about this. Participate in undergraduate research activities in the larger campus. You might want to go and help with research outside of nursing, for example, in psychology, social work, medicine, etc. More experienced practitioners have a greater advantage here because they can see the existing gaps in their current practice much more easily and identify areas for future research (Jolley, 2007).

Regardless of the level of education, focusing on one topic and elaborating this single topic demonstrates the applicants' vision and strategies to achieve this vision. These essays demonstrate who you are and where you stand from a scientific standpoint. Abstain from general statements such as "research is important because it solves major issues in healthcare" or "genetics allow us to identify pathways of disease" or "most behavioral nursing interventions are underutilized." Your answers should identify and reflect specific types of research that answer major research questions that you are passionate about. Why are you passionate about it? What methods best answer a specific question in your area of interest, and what do you already know about it? What type of behavioral interventions have shown efficacy in your area of interest, and how would you implement them? Because you have limited space for your essays, wasting it on general information that the reviewers already know will only weaken your application.

Letters of Recommendation

As the final part of an application to a PhD program, you must submit letters of recommendation. These letters come from professional colleagues, former professors, and other individuals who can provide strong statements about your professional and personal strengths and weaknesses.

These provide a fair outside judgment of whether you would be a good fit in a particular PhD program. So, carefully choose individuals who can make the best recommendation for you. Ask them before you select them as your recommenders whether they think they can give you a strong recommendation.

Often, applicants choose these individuals based on a favorite class in which they excelled or from among colleagues with whom they have worked in the past. Seriously consider selecting academic/professional leaders (professors, clinical instructors, charge nurses, nurse managers) as your recommenders; after all, they evaluate students/nurses on an ongoing basis. The person you select should be able to compare your skills and talents to those that they are currently dealing with. Again, if one of the people you had in mind for a recommendation letter does not feel comfortable giving you a strong recommendation, let it go; you do not make your application package stronger by going forward with that person.

TIP

Only choose people for your references who will give you the best reference ever. We strongly recommend not getting a lukewarm reference from a previous supervisor but rather get a strong reference from a direct colleague. That way your application goes forward with the strongest push towards an admission into a PhD program.

Ensuring a Positive PhD Training Experience

A positive PhD training experience depends on a number of factors that influence your advancement, including the following:

- Selecting the right mentor
- Taking the right coursework
- Involving yourself in ongoing research endeavors
- Joining a professional organization
- Planning your publication and dissemination efforts
- Planning a successful progression through your program

The following subsections explore these factors in more detail.

Selecting the Right Mentor

Identification of the right mentor starts by communicating with the faculty member who helped you with your application to the PhD program (Kim et al., 2009; Rodts & Lamb, 2008). If you still believe this is the best person to guide you in your first year, set up regular meetings.

TAILORING YOUR MENTORING EXPERIENCE

Joachim Voss

In my experience at the University of California, having had a mentor who requested weekly meetings with me was one of the great luxuries of my PhD training. I soon realized that I was the only PhD student in our cohort of 24 who had this arrangement of intensive mentoring during the first year. He requested that I come prepared with a question to talk about what I learned in class that week and to identify areas I struggled with. These 1-hour sessions allowed me to get to know my advisor and allowed him to get to know my scientific thinking. Our discussions shaped my theoretical thinking and the research approaches that I carried forward throughout the PhD program. Though it's not always the standard, this professor mentored me for my entire PhD program and well into my career. On the other hand, one-on-one weekly meetings may not work best for you.

Steven Simpkins

In my experience as a current PhD student, I prefer to meet less frequently with my mentor; perhaps three to four times a quarter. While we may not meet as often, our time is well-spent discussing classes and projects, planning for presentations and publications, and ensuring that I am on track both academically and emotionally. This has worked well for my mentor who is, of course, tremendously busy with his own work and his work with other students and has been effective for me and my tight schedule of activities and projects.

Selecting the Appropriate Coursework

Selection of the appropriate coursework includes program-specific core courses in sequence. Every class assignment should contribute, in the widest sense, to your future research topic (Kim et al., 2009). Selection of research methods classes (statistics, scale development, qualitative research methods, and so on) need to supplement the more conceptual and theoretical courses so that you gain a solid understanding of the various qualitative and quantitative measurement approaches that you can take in your research career.

> **TIP**
>
> *When taking these classes, use the research area you have in mind for the future in class assignments and projects. You can thus establish a great body of knowledge on your topic.*

Select courses that aid the focus of your future study within nursing and in fields adjacent to nursing (social work, medicine, global health, economics, sociology, and so forth); this will vary individually by topic and interest (Kim et al., 2009). As you proceed through your coursework, ask yourself whether your instructor would be a good advisor in you area of interest. If the answer is yes, speak to your advisor about that possibility.

Students often want to take more classes than feasible, either taking as many classes as possible each quarter or taking classes for 3 or 4 years. Both strategies serve only to delay the completion of your degree, and you might need to reevaluate what you are trying to accomplish. A PhD class load should never exceed 14 credits; otherwise, you do not have the time or the mental capacity to process the offered information, complete the required readings, or form solid opinions.

The first year of required classes represents an opportunity to learn how to think about research, your position in this new worldview, and to recognize your limitations. These classes provide you with boundaries with which you can continue to model the rest of your academic career. When you take more than four courses in a quarter or a semester, your workload becomes so high that you begin skimming the surface, never effectively penetrating the content. Focus instead on gaining in-depth knowledge of your area of research; only this approach will help you identify your knowledge/experience gaps (Jolley, 2007).

Taking courses for 3 or 4 years is an equally bad approach because many students lose interest in their topic and the identified scientific field will already have moved on from where they started 4 years earlier. Extending your coursework hampers your ability to enter the research arena with the most current knowledge, theory, and methods. Keeping your coursework to the planned 2 years ensures that you keep motivated, current, and moving forward with your cohort.

Involving Yourself in Ongoing Research Endeavors

From the beginning of your entry into the PhD program, pay attention to opportunities for taking research assistantships, joining research networks, becoming a member of professional nursing research organizations, and attending interprofessional research seminars. All these activities connect you to a professional network, alert you to funding opportunities (refer back to Table 9.1), and show you the reality of research-oriented faculty (Kim et al., 2006; Kim et al., 2009).

Faculty members in the research-intensive universities often seek PhD students to carry out aspects of their research. These research activities are usually paid, time limited, and provide you with an incredible opportunity to get an inside perspective of an established researcher's project with all its intricacies. Most important, these activities require tasks that you can learn quickly or that build upon existing strengths. A number of faculty members in your institution are involved in research networks, and these activities represent a unique chance to gain inside perspective of such networks.

NOTE

In his few years as a PhD student, Steven had many such opportunities. One particular activity was with an Return on Investment (ROI) research grant team as a research assistant. He was introduced to the principal investigator (PI) at a network event before he started his program

continues

and was able to hit the ground running from the start. Working with such a large study was invaluable in that it complemented his studies of how to conduct rigorous research, allowed him to work directly with clients as a data collector, and provided him a unique opportunity to be mentored by a collection of tenured researchers whom he might not have otherwise met had he not taken advantage of this opportunity.

Joining a Professional Organization

Each region in the United States has specialized nursing research societies that hold annual conferences, provide mentorship programs, offer grant money, and further research activities. Plan on joining a regional society and becoming an active member by serving among the leadership of such an organization or submitting a student poster. Examples might include, but are not limited to:

- American Thoracic Society: Nurses Section
- Association for Radiologic & Imaging Nursing
- Association of Child Neurology Nurses
- Association of Nurses in AIDS Care
- Association of Pediatric Oncology Nurses
- Association of periOperative Registered Nurses
- Association of Rehabilitation Nurses
- Association of Women's Health, Obstetric and Neonatal Nurses

Each state has either local chapters of those associations or special state-oriented nursing associations, and you can also get engaged in those.

Planning Your Publication and Dissemination Efforts

You and your mentor should carefully plan the activities that build your CV through national and international presentations and publications:

- An annual poster presentation at a regional research conference is an important first step in losing the initial stage fright.

- In your second year, you should be able to write a manuscript summarizing the current research literature in your area of interest (Williams & Jordan, 2007).

- In anticipation of starting data collection in year three, you begin the process of human subject approval, which can take months. In this time, you can write your next manuscript by evaluating your theoretical assumptions with existing frameworks detailing your theoretical thinking within the context of your area of interest.

- In the fourth or fifth year, after you have completed your data collection and data analysis, your next manuscript should be your first data-based publication. Much of this first manuscript exists already in your proposal, and you only need to include the results, discussion, and implication sections. Along the way, you will likely engage in research activities that result in publications at the end of the activity. Always get involved even if you are only a third, fourth, or fifth author.

Accomplishments such as these build up your CV and can help boost any postdoctoral position application (Jolley, 2007; Kim et al., 2009).

Planning a Successful Progression Through Your Program

Determining the right steps, monitoring your progress, and taking advice throughout the program at the right time are all part of your planning of the PhD (Williams & Jordan, 2007). A timetable with major milestones provides you and your mentor with a tool to evaluate your own progress. This plan includes the following:

- When to think about forming your committee

- When to begin the process for the general exams, when to apply for funding (refer again to Table 9.1)

- When to submit materials to the committee members

- When to have your proposal and your dissertation defense

It bears repeating that the role of open communication and sound planning between you and your mentor is critical in guiding all of these processes. These activities need to fit within the academic calendar of your respective institution and need to comply with the rules and regulations of the university.

The sooner you have your committee together, the sooner you can proceed with planning your exams and with your research project. Each potential committee member should represent one part of your dissertation topic. Each member should represent one of the following:

- Strength in the research topic

- Strength in theory development

- Strength in research methods

- An unbiased member outside the School of Nursing

- Your chair

You and your mentor will plan all the necessary steps for your general exam, communicate with the graduate school, monitor your progress, and ensure that the committee has approved your dissertation before you finalize and defend it.

Post-Doctorate Positions

Before you finish your PhD, you should get ready for the next step in your career: applying for and considering offers, accepting one, and then finally embarking on your first postdoctoral position.

> **NOTE**
>
> *Joachim finished his PhD program studying the predictors and correlates of fatigue in HIV. During the time he spent in the PhD program, he also had applied for a Green Card and worked for a Filipino temp agency. Two years into the PhD program he received his Green Card and was finally eligible (alien resident) to apply for grant funding from the U.S. government. While he was in full analysis mode for his dissertation, he found an incredible opportunity for postdoctoral training at the National Institutes of Health. With the help of a basic scientist (not his primary mentor), he applied and was accepted. Before he even defended his dissertation, he knew he would be moving to the East Coast, starting at the National Institutes of Health.*

A career in nursing research depends entirely on the ability of the individual to generate funding (refer again to Table 9.1), publish data-based manuscripts, engage students in your work, and be recognized for your accomplished work (Segrott, McIvor, & Green, 2006; Shirey, 2009). A postdoctoral phase for newly graduated PhDs usually guarantees them protected time to establish themselves and time to publish the rest of their PhD data. Most doctoral students have much more data than they can publish in one paper. This time also allows you to apply for money for your first independent research project without your PhD mentor.

Engagement in your new mentor's existing program of research makes the transition easier and provides you with opportunities to be involved with research and publications (Rodts & Lamb, 2008). This time is protected from all the requirements of a junior faculty member. Junior faculty members have requirements for teaching, service, and research; and these appointments often come with serious time commitments (Segrott et al., 2006). They often conduct research only on weekends or in the evenings after they have dealt with all the student issues, faculty meetings, committee memberships, and special projects.

If your personal and financial situations allow, enter a postdoctoral training period before you join a SON faculty. Postdoctoral positions can help you (although without guarantee) transition into that specific institution (Segrott et al., 2006). Repeat the same rigorous evaluation process that you performed for your PhD before you commit to a postdoctoral position. Again, you are committing resources, time, and energy, and you are asking another favor from your friends and family to support you through this phase.

Select a mentor for this phase of your career based on the mentor's ability to support your efforts in finding future employment, securing funding, disseminating your work at key nursing research conferences. You also want to ensure that your mentor can introduce you to deans and chairs of interested institutions (Edwards, Webber, Mill, Kahwa, & Roelofs, 2009; Rodts & Lamb, 2008).

Whether you stay or leave the current SON after your postdoctoral fellowship should depend on what you have accomplished and how much of your time you are able to protect in the first 2 years after becoming a junior faculty there (Segrott et al., 2006). Of course, the SON also needs to have a position open for which you can apply. All public institutions are required to have national searches for open positions, so having been a postdoctoral fellow at that institution does not guarantee that you will be the most qualified candidate. You need to be diligent and thorough in your approach to the application and interview process as though you were applying to a new institution.

Staying at the same institution has benefits and disadvantages. You know the place, have gotten to know some of the faculty, are aware of the current politics, and have a reasonable idea of what you can expect from the work environment. In addition, the faculty of the current SON knows both your strengths and weaknesses, you might not have funding (thus making you less competitive in a national search), and you might not like some aspects of the institution that much.

Going to a new place also has its pros and cons. On the one hand, you are a newcomer and the people who want to recruit you are motivated to get you to come there; therefore, you have more room for negotiation of the terms and conditions of your employment to get you there. On the other hand, you don't have any insights into the institution and its politics (good or bad).

> **NOTE**
>
> *In all honesty, there might never be a place where the institutional politics are completely friendly, the workload between the faculty distributed completely equally, or where the faculty all get along and respect each other. You might have to live with these imperfections and just be the best faculty member that you can be.*

Junior Faculty Positions

The day has come! You've signed on the dotted line and are now officially an assistant professor with tenure at a research-intensive university. You need to ensure that you have a good faculty mentor on your side to help you through the initial steps of junior faculty membership. You need to find someone who can connect you to the larger research community within the university, recommend school-wide committee activities that are not completely overwhelming, plan your progress toward your 3-year review, plan your first teaching engagements, and help you limit the amount of time you spend on service activities (Edwards et al., 2009; Rodts & Lamb, 2008). Let's elaborate on these steps.

Transitioning from a postdoctoral position to a new faculty position is a major shift. You must attend certain meetings in your department and in the school. Because of your expertise, you may have graduate students who want your mentorship and guidance for their PhD projects. You need money to sustain your new program of research and need time to develop grant proposals. You might be asked to lecture in classes or to be a co-teacher of a course. This can all be overwhelming and requires sufficient planning. Make a schedule and reserve time specifically for your research activities. Separate these time slots into actual research activities such as data collection, analysis, recruitment, laboratory activities, grant writing, preparations for human subject applications, manuscript writing, and other research-related writing.

In addition to your research schedule, find a regular day where you have open office hours for 2 to 3 hours for students so that they can schedule time to talk to you and seek your input. This will deter students from showing up randomly in your office during the week. Most schools have a day when much of the committee work is done. Following the recommendations of your mentor and your department chair, select a committee to sit on with a reasonable time commitment and stay with this committee for the first 3 years.

You also want to produce two or three manuscript submissions per year. This type of productivity pipeline gives you a sufficient record in terms of research for your 3-year promotion and tenure review (Williams & Jordan, 2007). Most institutions evaluate junior faculty annually within the school, in addition to a university evaluation after 3 years. The university thus evaluates your productivity and recommends strategies on how to strengthen your performance as you move toward your promotion and tenure review (Williams & Jordan, 2007).

Spend half of your first year on research activities such as grant writing to ensure that you have multiple grants in various stages of review and approval. In the current funding climate, the expectation of three to five grant applications a year does not underestimate the number of trials necessary to achieve success (Edwards et al., 2009; Rodts & Lamb, 2008). As mentioned earlier, you also want to prepare at least two or three publications during the first year. Doing so produces a pipeline of manuscripts at different stages: the planning stage, the writing phase, the review phase, the resubmission phase, and the publication phase. This approach ensures a continual record of dissemination.

A number of graduate students may seek you out as an advisor, so choose carefully only after speaking to their current advisors. Junior faculty members are often unaware of students who have had a number of advisors for various reasons. Choose wisely and make sure that you have matching interests.

NOTE

Never become a PhD committee member or a PhD chair because you feel sorry for a student. This does nothing for students to help them complete their program, nor does it help you to identify students who might work with you to build your research program.

For the first year, serving on one or two PhD committees will allow you to learn the rules of the university and how to conduct certain types of exams, meetings, and interactions between the students and their committee members (Williams & Jordan, 2007). During the first year, you also need to connect with your community members by joining a local chapter of nurses in a special disease association, by interacting with local providers, by engaging with research groups around campus, and by studying the cross-cutting funding opportunities (Edwards et al., 2009) (again, refer back to Table 9.1). By the end of your first year, you should feel more secure and respected for your accomplishments.

Even after you have successfully completed the requirements for your 3-year review with your department chair and your mentor, you want to continue moving your career forward. Slowly begin to build the momentum in your research career, increase your visibility in the science community, take on more national professional responsibilities, begin to be a reviewer for grant applications, seek opportunities to review journals, and begin to teach classes on a regular basis. In addition to your research, build your teaching portfolio with a sufficient number of peer and student evaluations (Williams & Jordan, 2007). Begin to look for more leadership training through the Robert Wood Johnson Foundation, the John A. Hartford Foundation, the Oncology Nursing Foundation, and other similar organizations. These types of programs require a 1- to 3-year commitment that focuses on your ability to lead change within your institution and beyond. Applications are highly competitive, and you and your mentor need to dedicate sufficient time to ensure strong science, strong personal documentation, and exceptional letters of support. You can find details on their websites, and requirements for application vary significantly.

You have now finished your leadership training. At this stage, you have likely gotten some larger grant funding, have published between 10 and 20 data-based papers, given lectures, and presented posters. You have probably received an award for your engagement in research, teaching, or service and have a portfolio of classes that you have taught and a number of graduate students who have graduated. You are ready for a promotion. Together, your chair and your mentor should now decide to submit you for tenure and promotion review.

At this point, you usually provide a summary of your current and anticipated research activities. You provide the same information about your teaching and service activities. You then have to verify this with letters of support from colleagues, mentees, and professional organizations that you have worked with who think highly of your engagement. Your package then goes out to senior faculty members of other institutions for an external review to determine whether you should be considered for promotion and tenure in their institution.

These reviews and your materials are then presented to your departmental Appointment and Tenure (APT) committee. All associate and full professors in the SON review your package and vote for it to move forward or not. You receive a letter from your chair that addresses how you can strengthen your package and rework any of your sections. If the vote is negative, the chair informs you and recommends a deferral. This means you have 1 more year to show additional improvement in an area identified as weak. After that year, you go through the process again, and your package has to go through the entire process regardless of the outcome of the department vote. Many of these details are specific to each institution, so read and understand the rules and regulations for promotion and tenure at the relevant institution.

Obviously, the shift from clinician to nurse researcher changes every aspect of your life. You need tenacity, a strong will to succeed, a lifelong curiosity, and a major dedication to train and educate others to follow in your footsteps. Securing and managing financial and human resources will become an important part of your daily life. Expert communication in meetings, on the phone, or by email requires different skills than those that you might have used successfully with your patients. You move from a status of colleague among peers on a unit or a clinic to a person of power for your students, a competitor for resources with your faculty colleagues, and a future leader within your institution or for other SONs. Along the way, you will find that your new scientific career is just as satisfying as your clinical work once was.

Finally, we wish for you to find the same excitement and passion that we have enjoyed during our research careers. No day in our lives has been like the day before, and our excitement has kept us coming back to our offices to start every day with enthusiasm for what we do: nursing research.

MEN IN NURSING RESEARCH SURVIVAL TIPS

Be prepared for competition at every step of your academic career.

Find a good match between you and your mentor's interests.

Choose a strong mentor for every stage of your academic career.

Stay focused and move along with enthusiasm.

Never forget to enjoy what you do.

Share your thoughts with your colleagues.

References

Edwards, N., Webber, J., Mill, J., Kahwa, E., & Roelofs, S. (2009). Building capacity for nurse-led research. *International Nursing Review, 56*, 88-94. doi:10.1111/j.1466-7657.2008.00683.x

Harding, T. (2009). Swimming against the malestream: Men choosing nursing as a career. *Nursing Praxis in New Zealand, 25*(3), 4-16.

Jolley, J. (2007). Choose your doctorate. *Journal of Clinical Nursing, 16*(2), 225-233. doi:10.1111/j.1365-2702.2006.01582.x

Kim, M. J., Holm, K., Gerard, P., McElmurry, B., Foreman, M., Poslusny, S., & Dallas, C. (2009). Bridges to a doctorate: Mentored transition to successful completion of doctoral study for underrepresented minorities in nursing science. *Nursing Outlook, 57*(3), 166-171. doi:10.1016/j.outlook.2009.01.004

Kim, M. J., McKenna, H. P., & Ketefian, S. (2006). Global quality criteria, standards, and indicators for doctoral programs in nursing; literature review and guideline development. *International Journal of Nursing Studies, 43*, 477-489. doi:10.1016/j.ijnurstu.2005.07.003

Kjellgren, K. I., Welin, C., & Danielson, E. (2005). Evaluation of doctoral nursing programs: A review and a strategy for follow up. *Nurse Education Today, 25*(4), 316-325. doi:10.1016/j.nedt.2005.02.002

Lou, J. H., Yu, H. Y., & Chen, S. H. (2010). Factors affecting the career development of male nurses: A structural equation model. *Journal of Advanced Nursing, 66*(4), 900-910. doi:10.1111/j.1365-2648.2010.05264.x

Marsland, L., & Hickey, G. (2003). Planning a pathway in nursing: Do course experiences influence job plans? *Nursing Education Today, 23*(3), 226-235. doi:10.1016/S0260-6917(02)00196-X

Meachin, K., & Webb, C. (1996). Training to do women's work in a man's world. *Nursing Education Today, 16*(3), 180-188. PII:S0260-6917(96)80021-9

Nehls, N., & Barber, G. (2011). A prebaccalaureate PhD option: Shaping the future of research-focused doctoral education. *Educational Innovations, 51*(1), 50-53. doi:10.3928/01484834-20111116-06

Rodts, M. F., & Lamb, K. V. (2008). Transforming your professional self: Encouraging lifelong personal and professional growth. *Orthopaedic Nursing, 27*(2), 125-132. doi:10.1097/01.NOR.0000315628.45923.33

Segrott, J., McIvor, M., & Green, B. (2006). Challenges and strategies in developing nursing research capacity: A review of the literature. *International Journal of Nursing Studies, 43*(5), 637-651. doi:10.1016/j.ijnurstu.2005.07.011

Shields, L., Hall, J., & Mamun, A. A. (2011). The 'gender gap' in authorship in nursing literature. *Journal of the Royal Society in Medicine, 104*(11), 457-464. doi:10.1258/jrsm.2011.110015

Shirey, M. R. (2009). Building an extraordinary career in nursing: Promise, momentum, and harvest. *The Journal of Continuing Education in Nursing, 40*(9), 394-400. doi:10.3928/00220124-20090824-01

Williams, M., & Jordan, K. (2007). The nursing professional portfolio: A pathway to career development. *Journal for Nurses in Staff Development, 23*(3), 125-131. doi:10.1097/01.NND.0000277181.24959.3b

Chapter 10
Evolving Awareness

Daniel J. Pesut, PhD, RN, PMHCNS-BC, FAAN, ACC
Professor of Nursing Population Health and Systems
Cooperative Unit
Director, Katharine J. Densford International Center
for Nursing Leadership
Katherine R. and C. Walton Lillehei Chair in Nursing Leadership
University of Minnesota School of Nursing

> "We journey inward to know ourselves so we may take better charge of our lives, act more consciously, and be less motivated and driven by unconscious needs, desires, and powers."
> —William Miller (1989, p.27)

Men in nursing will find many of the topics addressed in this book valuable. For example, you must know how to navigate career aspirations, how to focus and choose a special area of practice, and how to lead in complex organizations. You must have a skill set to navigate the complexities of politics and the business of caring. You have a social responsibility to address issues of discrimination, diversity, and gender imbalance/balance. However, through all of this, you also don't want to forget to attend to the hard work of personal, psychological, and spiritual integration.

A journey toward personal, psychological, and spiritual integration is supported by the adoption of integral life practice (ILP). "Integral life practices are ways of organizing the many practices handed down through the centuries along with those practices developed at the cutting edge of psychology, consciousness studies, and other leading fields using a framework optimized for life in the 21st century" (Wilber, Patten, Leonard, & Morelli, 2008, p. 1). The four core modules of integral life practice relate to body, mind, spirit, and shadow (http://www.integral-life-practice.com). This chapter describes an ILP worldview and how to work through the intrapersonal dynamics associated with interpersonal shadow projections.

A journey toward integration requires mastery and management of yourself, mastery of communication, mastery of relationships, and mastery of multiple ways of being, thinking, feeling, and doing. The journey toward integration requires attention to multiple lines of intelligence and development: mind, body, spirit, and shadow work. Men who practice nursing should attend to this integration because integral life practice supports self-awareness and balance. Integral life practice supports the development of resilience, and when we care for ourselves, we are better equipped to care for others with intention and integrity.

Personal and Professional Notes

Personally speaking, nursing as a career has been a means for personal, psychological, and spiritual integration. I was attracted to nursing as a professional career for several reasons. First, nursing is a healing art and science. Second, I get bored very easily, and nursing is never boring and offers tremendous options for different career paths within one discipline. Third, nursing is consistent with the service and care orientation (people at the center) that my life path is about. Nursing focuses on very intimate human responses to illness and injury and the professional care required to help people manage and navigate those responses. I am and have always been most interested in psychological health and spiritual integration rather than disease and illness.

I enjoy the complexity and intellectual challenge of nursing. I think nursing entails six logics:

- The logic of the person needing care

- The logic of the nursing care problems people have to deal with

- The logic of the care planning process

- The logic of the relationships and complexity of nursing care issues

- The logic, limitations, and resources of the system in which one works

- The logic of managing and monitoring oneself

Managing yourself requires dealing with personal and professional interpersonal dynamics, some of which you might deem positive and some more challenging. When you encounter negative or positive disturbances in the environment, you have an invitation to engage in shadow work. Such shadow work is a journey toward integration.

DEFINING YOUR SHADOW WORK

Miller (1981) proposes this exercise as one way to tap into one's shadow: Think of someone you dislike. List all the qualities you do not like in that person (perhaps control, egocentrism, arrogance, defensiveness, sarcasm, clinging behavior, dependency). These identified qualities seed your shadow work. For what we often dislike in others are really qualities we ourselves possess, and we might not even be aware that we possess them.

Throughout my years as a clinician, consultant, educator, and coach I have had a keen interest in learning and helping people focus on purpose, strengths, and talents in an integral way. Helping people develop personal insight and skills and the ability to negotiate difficult conversations and difficult people is a leadership skill set. I believe that insight and understanding of one's purpose, strengths, and shadow issues is a prerequisite to the development and understanding of how best to lead, influence, grow, and develop in any context. Becoming more conscious of one's thoughts, feelings, beliefs, and projections is an invitation for personal growth and professional development. Inner work (attending to issues of archetypes, symbols, and shadow) is one way to help people heal into the future (Pesut, 2001, 2007).

In his study of ordinary people who achieve extraordinary change, Quinn (2000) notes the following commonalities among effective leaders:

- They envisioned productive community.
- They looked within.
- They embraced the hypocritical self.
- They transcended fear.
- They embodied a vision of the common good.
- They disturbed the system.
- They surrendered to the emergent process.
- They enticed through moral power.
- They accomplished the extraordinary.

Each of the leaders Quinn discusses pursued the good life while negotiating and managing fears and embracing the dark and light sides of themselves in a generative way. I believe extraordinary leaders develop an appreciation for an integral view of life and embrace shadow work as a means to embrace the hypocritical self and transcend fear. Such personal and professional responsibility supports a vision of the common good and often does disturb the system, thus resulting in a greater good.

Integral Theory and Integral Life Practice

Integral theory is emerging as a new conceptual framework that supports human development and provides a blueprint for the inner journey toward personal, psychological, and spiritual integration. Wilber (2000, 2001, 2005, 2007), a philosopher-scientist-practitioner, has advanced an integrally informed approach to being and doing in the world. *Integral* means comprehensive, balanced, whole, and complete. For an excellent overview and introduction to integral theory, see Esbjorn-Hargens's (n.d.) Integral Life website (http://integrallife.com/node/37539).

WHY ARE INTEGRAL LIFE PRACTICES IMPORTANT?

Integral life practices include and integrate three kinds of health (Wilber et al., 2008). Horizontal health is the dynamic fulfillment of the possibilities for awareness, aliveness, and care available to each person at their current level of development. Vertical health is growth into greater conscious awareness and complexity. As you grow vertically, you transcend and include past developmental ways of being and move upward toward new stages of development. Essential health involves recognition and appreciation for mystery and spirit in your life. I believe it is essential for all nurses to engage in "inner work" that supports outer service and personal, psychological, and spiritual growth, development, and integration (Pesut, 2001).

According to Forman (2010), integral philosophy involves attention to the following principles:

- *What is real and important depends on your perspective.*

continues

- *Everyone is at least partially right about what he argues is real and important.*

- *By bringing together these partial perspectives, you can construct a more complete and useful set of truths.*

From an integral philosophy, a person's perspective depends on five central things:

- *The way the person gains knowledge (the person's primary perspective, tools, or discipline)*

- *The person's level of identity development*

- *The person's level of development in other key domains or lines*

- *The person's particular state at any given time*

- *The person's personality style or "type" (cultural and gender style)*

The integral viewpoint is often relayed using the acronym AQAL, which stands for all quadrants, all levels (or all lines/states or all types). The AQAL model provides a map for the development of integral consciousness that embraces the importance and value of shadow work.

The AQAL Model's Four Quadrants

Four major overarching perspectives (quadrants) can be described using the AQAL model, which provides a framework for most of life. Personal development and evolution within the context of the AQAL framework is about harmonizing development across all four quadrants (see Figure 10.1) to reach more integrated levels of development:

- **I:** The first dimension is one's individual interior: one's thoughts, feelings, intentions, and psychology. Basically, this is the I of you.

- **We:** The second quadrant refers to your collective interior (your relationships, culture, and meaning that you share with others). This quadrant is often referred to as the We space.

- **It:** The third quadrant is an individual's individual exterior. This individual exterior is one's physical body and behaviors and actions. This is referred to as the It space.

- **Its:** Finally, there is the quadrant of one's collective exterior. This is the environment and social systems and structures in which an individual operates. This is referred to as the Its space.

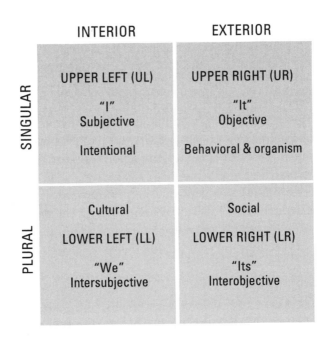

FIGURE 10.1

Four quadrants of the AQAL model.

Figure from Sherwood & Horton-Deutsch, 2012

I Space

Consider and reflect on your experience in this moment using the quadrants as a map. Tune inward into awareness of your sense of self. This I space consists of thoughts, ideas, opinions, motivations, values, beliefs, and a sense of identity purpose, mission, and vision. All of these exist within the interior of your personal consciousness. All of these things are invisible to those around you; they are available only to you. You might study these aspects of your own experience through the use of journaling, prayer, self-inquiry, mindfulness practices, meditation, reflection, or phenomenology. What you know about yourself depends on your sincerity of expression, truthfulness, honesty, integrity, and your willingness to acknowledge your biases and identify your assumptions and experiences. Self-knowledge influences how you see the world and thus begins the sense-making of practice, work, and relationships with others.

We Space

Next, stop for a moment and think about one of your relationships. Imagine partnering with another person. You communicate with this person, share emotions, share feelings, and participate in the ups and downs of relating. The feeling and awareness of the We you get from this relationship is different from the awareness of I. What you know about the We often derives from resonance and mutual understanding, empathy, collective reflection, storytelling, and dialogue/debate.

It Space

The It space refers to the perspective or dimension of objectifying people and things and sensing behaviors. This is the dimension of individual exteriors. This is the dimension of body and brain: You can see it, hear it, touch it, taste it, and smell it. The focus on the exterior individual nature of something gives it a "thingness" sense. You can study the dimension of it through observations and measures from the outside in: controlled conditions, representative samples, empirical measures, fieldwork observations, surveys, documentation, and examinations. It is often described in third-person descriptions and supported with statistics and charts. Physical behavior and the things one does with the body are a part of the It dimension because others can see and observe these behaviors and actions.

Its Space

Now consider the Its dimension. The Its dimension involves the social and political systems in which you live and work. This includes the environment, the ecology of the planet, the social systems of schools, and the government. It encompasses policies and procedures that regulate your work and family life, as well as the legal system in which you participate. Its awareness includes experiences with multiple interacting systems that focus on function and sustainability and the ecology of the planet and local environment where you live and work.

Integral philosophy supports people who aspire to ILPs (Wilber et al., 2008) and who recognize these four different dimensions of awareness are co-arising at the same time. None of the dimensions exist separately, yet we often segregate and discuss them one at a time, as if the one dimension does not influence the other dimensions. Integral philosophy and theory challenges us to be aware of the four dimensions in an intentional way. Such awareness sharpens our intention and attention and provides us with alternative ways to investigate phenomena while appreciating and valuing multiple perspectives in the pursuit of learning, inquiry, and knowledge. In this way, we expand our reflective capacity and journey inward toward new insights, appreciation, and integration of our complexities that include levels and lines of development as well as states of awareness we experience and the types of people we are.

For example, levels provide you one way to describe developmental structures that evolve over time. As you grow and mature, you evolve through developmental stages. A pattern of development evolves from an egocentric view of the world, to an ethnocentric one, and then a world-centric stage of development often becomes evident over time.

Lines

A line refers to a specific area of growth and development. For example, important lines of development and life questions include the following:

- **Cognitive:** What am I aware of?
- **Self:** Who am I?
- **Values:** What is significant to me?
- **Moral:** What should I do?
- **Interpersonal:** How should we interact?
- **Spiritual:** What is of ultimate concern?
- **Needs:** What do I need?
- **Kinesthetic:** How should I physically do this?
- **Emotional:** How do I feel about this?
- **Aesthetic:** What is attractive to me?

Lines of development arise in any of the four quadrants. For example, some lines of development in the I quadrant are cognitive awareness, emotional access, interpersonal skills, psychosexual expression, moral capacity, spiritual experience, and self-identity dynamics.

Lines of development in the We quadrant are such things as worldviews, intersubjective dynamics, linguistic meaning, cultural values, background cultural contexts, philosophical positions, and religious understandings.

Lines of development in the It quadrant include organic structures, neuronal systems, neurotransmitters, brainwave patterns, skeletal-muscular growth, nutritional intake, and kinesthetic capacity.

Examples of lines of development in the Its quadrant include geopolitical structures, ecosystems, written legal codes, architectural styles, grammatical systems, evolutionary paths.

States

From an integral perspective, states matter. States in the integral framework are temporary, changing levels of awareness. Consider how you personally transition every day from dreaming to sleeping to waking states. People can also alter their states through meditating or exercising. Some people have psychic state experiences; others alter their states through the use of chemicals or substances. So, in the I quadrant you find phenomenal states, natural states, and altered states. In the We quadrant, you find group states, intersubjective states, and religious states. In the It quadrant, you find brain states, hormonal states, and behavioral states. In the Its quadrant, you find weather states, economic states, and ecological states.

Types

In the integral model, the notion of types represents another basic building. These are categories of differences like masculine or feminine, cultural types, or personality types like Myers-Briggs personality definitions that become influential as you think about integral paths of growth and development through time. So, in the I quadrant, you can reference personality and gender types. In the We quadrant, you can reference types of religious and kinship systems. In the It quadrant, you can reference blood types and body types. In the Its quadrant, types include biome types and regime types.

Using the AQAL Model

A person can use the AQAL model to assess any situation. For example, different situations challenge you individually, so you have *interior considerations* as well as *interpersonal communications* that pose challenges to you in terms of evaluating possible *actions to take*. And the influence of your actions has a reciprocal relationship impacting *systems* in which you operate. It is easy to visualize the challenges in teamwork communication, an essential aspect of quality and safety, within these considerations of the four quadrants.

Imagine that the four quadrants represent a circle. To have an integral perspective means that you pay attention to all four quadrants and all 360 degrees of the circle. To limit your attention or awareness to only one of the quadrants means that you are attending to only 90 degrees of what is tetra-arising or possible at any given moment. ILPs and shadow work require 360 degrees of awareness. Each moment, you can ask the following questions to develop a 360-degree integral awareness:

- **Engage in Integral Scan:** What do I think, feel, or value about _____? (Focus on I, the interior individual.)

- **Communication:** How can I take the greatest number of people into consideration at the deepest levels? (Focus on We, the collective interior of relationships and relating.)

- **Evaluate possible actions:** What creative action can I take ____? (Focus on It, the exterior individual behavior and actions.)

- **Interconnections:** How do the larger systems in which I live affect my range of choices? How will my choices affect these systems? (Focus on Its, the collective exterior systems.)

Integral awareness helps you expand your notion of the world and your place in it. Integral consciousness also provides a means to develop all the essential elements in the AQAL model. For example, exercising different perspectives helps you appreciate the complexities of situations and events. Attending to your body strengthens and supports your energy, stamina, and ability to maintain optimum health. Attending to the spirit and community helps you navigate the complexities of meaning-making and community engagement in service of a professional purpose. Many modules are embedded in ILPs, but the one I have found most useful relates to shadow work.

Journeying Toward Integration

A paradox I have come to accept is how my dislike, discomfort, criticism, or outrage/anger with someone is really more about me than the person who is the object of my feelings (either positive or negative). I now realize through ILP and shadow work that what I most dislike or admire in someone is really an aspect of myself that I dislike or admire. Negative qualities are dark shadows. But the same dynamic of noting positive qualities in others may reveal our golden shadows. What we admire in others, in fact, are qualities that we possess in ourselves.

Until recently, there has not been a focus on shadow work outside of therapeutic circles. Richo writes, "The shadow is the archetype of the unconscious that represents the feared, denied, and unaddressed, forbidden and excluded parts of ourselves" (1991, p. 93):

- The negative shadow relates to those things that we are unconscious of in ourselves and that we disown and consequently recognize and condemn in others.

- The positive shadow refers to those things that we admire and perhaps envy in others that in fact are our own good qualities that we disavow in ourselves.

(Richo, 1991)

Miller writes that:

> "...*only he who is substantially conscious of the light should journey into his darkness. For the darkness will convict him and seek to destroy him and only the light can save him. Therefore we seek more light, more goodness, more moral strength and stamina when we make friends with our shadow. For that we must do, no matter what.*" *(1981, p. 142)*

Shadow work is an ILP that involves an inner journey of moving away from a neurotic ego conditioned by fear to building a healthy ego through inner work and integrating and containing all of one's hopes, fears, desires (Richo, 1991).

Most of the challenges I have faced as a male in nursing relate to balancing paradox, negotiating polarities, integrating and reconciling opposite or discordant qualities, and confronting the negative and positive aspects of shadow. The complementary nature of conscious-unconscious often manifests in interpersonal dynamics. Sometimes, we are conscious of our thoughts and feelings toward others, and other times we are not so conscious. When we are upset or disturbed by others, we are really tapping into unacknowledged instincts, motivations, and values of our own.

Over time, I have learned that thinking and reasoning about people, processes, and interpersonal dynamics as contrary or opposite often leads to polarized debate and discourse, to either-or, right-wrong thinking and reasoning. I find that we seldom consider or recognize the complementary nature of our projections and the value inherent, the personal growth and professional insights we can find, in reflecting on and processing our projections. The journey toward integration requires shadow work.

Shadow work is essential to personal and professional integration (Barry & Blanford, 1999; Egan, 1994; Richo, 1991).

Miller (1989) suggests that five effective paths exist for traveling inward to gain shadow insights:

- Soliciting feedback from others as to how they perceive us

- Uncovering the content of our projections

- Examining our behavior and exploring what is really occurring when we are perceived other than we intend to be perceived

- Considering our humor and identifications

- Studying our dreams, daydreams, and fantasies

The following several examples highlight practices that support working the shadow side as you journey toward integration through inner work. Engaging in shadow work is a choice, and people can work toward owning their own shadow, realize the shadow dynamic, and process it in an integral way. Otherwise, people may end up being owned by a shadow, where disowned feelings, drives, motivations, and beliefs shape their lives in unconscious ways. As quoted at the beginning of the chapter, Miller observes, "We journey inward to know ourselves so we may take better charge of our lives, act more consciously, and be less motivated and driven by unconscious needs, desires, and powers" (1989, p. 27).

3-2-1 ILP Shadow Process

The reality is that many people do not want to see their shadow and deal with the deep introspection and honesty that comes with working the shadow side of their personality. It takes a special kind of work to address personal shadow issues. Ford (1998) suggests that our shadows can teach us, guide us, and give us the blessing of being our entire self. If we journey inward toward integration, shadows are resources for us to expose and explore.

One core ILP is the 3-2-1 shadow process. For a description of the 3-2-1 shadow process, listen to Diane Hamilton at http://www.youtube.com/watch?v=x64raziI_4I

- The 3 in the 3-2-1 process is observing and noticing the positive or negative disturbance that you experience with someone. Describe the disturbance in as much detail as possible, keeping the description in the third person (he, him, she, her, they, their, it, its).

- Next, in the 2 phase of the 3-2-1 process, start a dialogue with the disturbance. Talk directly to the person, situation, or image, posing questions: Who or what are you? What do you want from me? What do you need to tell me? This is second person relating to the disturbance. Gain as much information as you can from the dialogue.

- Then move to the 1 of the 3-2-1 process. I, first person. Be the disturbance you have witnessed and related to. See the world and yourself as this disturbance and a part of you. Acknowledge that the disturbance is in fact a part of you (dark or golden shadow).

Pay attention to how this process shifts your perspective and your reaction to the other person and or disturbances in the environment. The 3-2-1 shadow ILP provides you a strategy to face, talk to, and be the shadow that you project toward others.

Befriending the Light and Dark of Shadow

Richo (1991) suggests a three-step process to befriend the positive side of the personal shadow:

1. Affirm that you have the quality you admire in someone else.

2. Act as if you have that quality by making choices that demonstrate it.

3. Announce to others that you are making these changes and enacting the positive quality and invite them to support your affirmation and actions in regard to the quality.

In contrast, Richo (1991) suggests a five-step process for befriending the negative personal shadow:

1. Acknowledge the fact that you have all the attributes that humans are capable of exhibiting, both the negative and positive aspects of a complementary pair.

2. Allow yourself to hold and cradle these parts of yourself. Acknowledge that they may have gone underground for a purpose or reason and may be turned into something more creative and useful in your life.

3. Admit to yourself and at least one other person these shadow insights and discoveries about yourself.

4. Make amends to those who may have been hurt by your personal denial of your own shadow parts.

5. Become aware of the kernel of value in your negative shadow and treat it as a positive shadow opportunity: affirm, act, and announce.

Consider practicing this exercise adapted from Richo's work on how to befriend the shadow. Study the characteristics listed in the left column of Table 10.1 that are often projected onto others. Each of these qualities has a complementary opposite that is listed in the right column.

TABLE 10.1 Working the Shadow Side

PROJECTED	UNOWNED
If you are strongly upset by others'...	Then you have but might not be using your own...
Addictiveness	Steadfastness
Anxiety	Excitement
Approval seeking	Openness to appreciation
Arrogance	Self-confidence
Bias	Discernment
Bitterness, grudge-holding	Refusal to overlook injustice
Caretaking	Compassion
Clinging	Loyalty
Conning	Teaching, encouraging
Control, manipulativeness	Leadership, efficiency, coordinating ability
Cruelty	Anger
Defensiveness	Preparedness
Demanding	Asking
Guilt	Conscientiousness
Incompetence	Willingness to experiment
Indecision	Openness to possibilities
Loneliness	Open to nurturance
Neediness	Asks for respect of appropriate needs
Perfectionism	Commitment to do things well
Procrastination	Commitment to do things in a timely way
Sarcasm	Wit
Self-pity	Self-forgiveness
Sense of obligation	Choice
Tactless bluntness	Frank candidness
Taking for granted	Accepting
Vengeful	Justice

Adapted from Richo, 1991, pp. 95-97.

Use the following method to work with the negative shadow and integrate the positive shadow qualities in the column on the right (RC) that are complementary to the projected negative shadow qualities in the column on the left (LC):

- I am strongly upset when others are _____. (Pick a projected negative quality from the LC.)

- I acknowledge that I am _____ (insert the projected negative quality from the LC) although I might not see it right now.

- I have _____ (insert the unowned contrasted positive quality from the RC) that I have not fully used.

- I choose to act if I have a high level of _____ (the positive quality from the RC) without being _____ (the negative quality from the LC).

The purposes of this chapter were to introduce integral theory and integral life practices (ILP) as a model and method for personal development and professional well-being, discuss the concept of shadow work as a key ILP, promote shadow work as a strategy to gain personal insight into professionally challenging relationship dynamics, and explain strategies and techniques that support shadow work in the context of ILP. Although you have many issues to navigate as a male in nursing, perhaps the most challenging is the journey toward integration and managing one's self. ILPs provide a blueprint for action and a roadmap for developing integral consciousness and life practices that support evolution and development through time.

People come into our lives for reasons, an idea integral to Rosen's four premises in *Thank You for Being Such a Pain*:

- Life's random encounters and people we meet are not so random after all.

- The pain, frustration, and joy we experience with other people are just as important for our personal, psychological, and spiritual growth as love and joy. Adversity is our teacher pushing past our resistance and teaching us what we would otherwise fail to learn.

- Difficult relationships can and should be healed because learning how to transform enmity is one of our most important life lessons.

- Healing requires being attentive to the spiritual lessons life presents us; when we do the inner work we are here to do, our outer relationships and circumstances become transformed.

(Rosen, 1998)

The people we encounter in our lives, whether they are colleagues or patients, provide us with opportunities to learn and grow. Sometimes we may defend ourselves against those we do not like or who rub us the wrong way. A fundamental premise of the shadow work in this chapter is that such a reaction is not really about the "other" person. Positive or negative reactions that we have toward others are really invitations to learn more about ourselves. Shadow work is a process that supports this learning and helps us grow, develop and evolve—personally, professionally, and spiritually.

MEN IN NURSING SURVIVAL TIPS

Personal, psychological, and spiritual integration is just as important for male nurses as coursework and clinical practice.

Person-to-person encounters, both positive and negative, are learning opportunities.

Becoming aware of, and actively working through, shadow issues promotes professional success and prevents professional derailment.

References

Barry, C., & Blanford, M. E. (1999). Shadow work seminars. 13706 Buckhorn Rd., Loveland, Colorado, 80538. Telephone 970-203-0400 or on the web at http://www.shadowwork.com

Egan, G. (1994). *Working the shadow side: A guide to positive behind-the-scenes management.* San Francisco, CA: Jossey-Bass.

Esbjorn-Hargens, S. (n.d.). An overview of integral theory: An all-inclusive framework for the 21st century. Integral Life Institute. Retrieved from http://integrallife.com/node/37539 (also available as Integral Institute, Resource Paper No. 1, March 2009)

Ford, D. (1998). *The dark side of the light chasers: Reclaiming your power, creativity, brilliance, and dreams.* New York, NY: Riverhead Books.

Forman, M. D. (2010). *A guide to integral psychotherapy.* Albany, NY: State University of New York (SUNY) Press.

Miller, W. A. (1981). *Make friends with your shadow: How to accept and use positively the negative side of your personality.* Minneapolis, MN: Augsburg Fortress.

Miller, W. A. (1989). *Your golden shadow: Discovering and fulfilling your undeveloped self.* San Francisco, CA: Harper and Row.

Pesut, D. J. (2001). Healing into the future: Re-creating the profession of nursing through inner work. In N. Chaska (Ed.), *The Nursing Profession: Tomorrow and Beyond* (pp. 853-867). Thousand Oaks, CA: Sage.

Pesut, D. J. (2007). Leadership: How to achieve success in nursing organizations. In C. O'Lynn & R. Tranbarger (Eds.), *Men in Nursing: History, Challenges and Opportunities* (pp. 153-168). New York, NY: Springer Publishing.

Quinn, R. E. (2000). *Change the world: How ordinary people can accomplish extraordinary results.* San Francisco, CA: Jossey-Bass.

Richo, D. (1991). *How to be an adult: A handbook on psychological and spiritual integration.* Mahwah, NJ: Paulist Press.

Rosen, M. I. (1998). *Thank you for being such a pain: Spiritual guidance for dealing with difficult people.* New York, NY: Three Rivers Press.

Sherwood, G., & Horton-Deutsch, S. (2012). *Reflective practice: Transforming education and improving outcomes.* Indianapolis, IN: Sigma Theta Tau International.

Wilber, K. (2000). *Integral psychology: Consciousness, spirit, psychology, therapy.* Boston, MA: Shambala Press.

Wilber K. (2001). *A theory of everything: An integral vision for business, politics, science and spirituality.* Boston, MA: Shambala Press.

Wilber, K. (2005). Introduction to integral theory and practice: IOS basic and the AQAL map. *AQAL: Journal of Integral Theory and Practice, 1*(1), 1-36.

Wilber, K. (2007). *The integral vision: A very short introduction to the revolutionary integral approach to life, God, the universe, and everything.* Boston, MA: Shambala Press.

Wilber, K., Patten, T., Leonard, A., & Morelli, M. (2008). *Integral life practice: A 21st century blueprint for physical health, emotional balance, mental clarity, and spiritual awakening.* Boston, MA: Integral Books.

Chapter 11

Intrapreneuring: Thoughts on Nurses Leaving or Staying in the Business World

Roy L. Simpson, DNP, RN, DPNAP, FAAN
Vice President Nursing, Cerner Corporation
Kansas City, Missouri

An often misunderstood concept, the term *intrapreneuring* simply refers to acting as an entrepreneur inside a larger organization. A deceptively simple approach on paper, intrapreneurship actually demands that those employed with larger organizations possess the passion, competencies, and attitude needed to wholeheartedly engage in their reinvention (Pinchot, 1985). The widespread consolidation making its way through the ranks of America's health care organizations suggests that now is the time for nurses to take a long look at their current roles, responsibilities, and futures.

In his landmark intrapreneuring treatise, Pinchot laid out 10 basic tenets that drive intrapreneurship:

1. Come to work each day willing to be fired.

2. Circumvent any orders aimed at stopping your dream.

3. Do any job needed to make your project work, regardless of your job description.

4. Find people to help you.

5. Follow your intuition about the people you choose, and work only with the best.

6. Work underground as long as you can; publicity triggers the corporate immune system.

7. Never be in a race unless you are running in it.

8. Remember, it is easier to ask for forgiveness than for permission.

9. Be true to your goals, but be realistic about the ways to achieve them.

10. Honor your sponsors.

(Pinchot, 1985, p. 22)

Recently, Pinchot added the following "commandments" to his original 10:

1. Ask for advice before asking for resources.

2. Express gratitude.

3. Build your team; intrapreneuring is not a solo activity.

4. Share credit widely.

5. Keep the best interests of the company and its customers in mind when you have to bend the rules or circumvent the bureaucracy.

6. Don't ask to be fired; even as you bend the rules and act without permission, use all the political skill you and your sponsors can muster to move the project forward without making waves.

(Pinchot, 2011)

Every nurse in America could benefit by taking what Pinchot says to heart, not just men. For those of you with a history in nursing, can you say that you are as engaged in the profession as you were when you started? If not, it might be time for a bit of reinvention. For those of you picking up speed, what is holding you back? Again, some of Pinchot's advice may resonate with you. Wherever in nursing you find yourself today, you won't be there much longer. The industry consolidation, the pressure to perform, and the payment squeeze are all collaborating to change health care as we know it today.

As you mull your future, understand that what Pinchot means is that every choice is a choice (even if you are choosing to do nothing). Effective choices made inside the organization and outside it demand that the chooser be cognizant not only of the immediate and short-term rewards, benefits, and consequences of the choice but also of the long-range impacts.

With all due respect to Pinchot, nurses need 10 additional tenets to live and thrive inside their organizations. Each of these recommendations springs from an actual event or series of events that occurred in a clinical or corporate organization. The names of those involved have been removed so as to offer these suggestions anonymously.

1. **Be aware that corporate reorganizations are designed to benefit those who orchestrate them, not the participants.** Of course, participants often benefit from such realignments, but these "happy circumstances" are merely unintended byproducts of the reorganization. Consider this example: An executive nurse with more than 30 years of

experience in the organization was assured by
her incoming superior that she could continue
overseeing the nursing organization post-acquisition.
Despite these assurances, she wisely asked her
current superior to write into her employment
contract that if she were released within the 12
months following the acquisition she would receive
18 months' pay. Just 7 weeks later, she lost her job.

Mergers and acquisitions are financial transactions
that affect people, but the business reasons behind
mergers and acquisitions trump the human capital
side of the equation every time. To understand a
business combination, look beyond the publicity and
hype to understand why the transaction makes sense
and who is really "winning here." If you are with
the acquiring company, you won. If you are with
the company being acquired, life as you know it is
over. All the leverage stays with the acquiring side
of the transaction. That's where the power is, and
that's where the decisions will be made. You might
be asked for your opinion or recommendation, but
don't count on it being followed.

2. **Know what the position requires before you
    accept it.** These days, many people start their own
    businesses because they assume (some rightly, some
    not) that because they are good at their current
    job they can make a business of it. Unfortunately,
    this is often not the case. Owning and operating a
    business requires a range of skills, from strategic
    planning and marketing to financial and operational
    competencies, that most budding entrepreneurs find
    baffling (Gerber, 1995). Recognize the fact that most
    human beings are short on vision and acknowledge
    that selling a product that exists is easier and
    quicker than selling a concept that may exist only

in your own mind. If you are terminated (with or without cause), know what you agree to when you sign those termination papers. Read the termination agreement line for line. If you don't understand the language, don't sign. Consult a labor attorney who can interpret them for you, and then decide whether to sign. Hiring an attorney to represent your position in a nonemotional way can often effect a better outcome than you can negotiate for yourself.

3. **Acknowledge that every question has more than one answer and every choice has more than two options.** At its essence, no choice really comes down to A versus B; there's always C, D, and M to consider as well. Don't ignore the often-overlooked expense of lost opportunities. What could you be doing other than the thing you are doing now, and what would be the result of doing that other thing? For example, you may expect your employer to do business in a certain way. However, the company might elect to operate in a different way for economic reasons. Because executives see the choice as a clearly economic one, they might apply little logic in the decision-making. For example, corporations often elect to write a check to silence an employee passed over for promotion rather than fight a discrimination case. In another instance, which appears similar on the surface, the board and executive team may choose to take an individual on legally to stop that person from joining a competitor. Unless you know the situation from both sides, you won't likely see the difference in the two scenarios, which, from the outside, look similar.

4. **Understand that every waking moment and thought you have becomes intellectual property owned by**

your employer, not by you. This tenet holds true for every human being on the planet who endorses a payroll check (unless you have an idea totally unlinked, unassociated, uninfluenced, or untied to your employment). For example, the nurse leader who starts a bait-and-tackle shop is probably in the clear. That said, some academic institutions have very different ways of valuing intellectual property. So, understand who owns what in your environment. Again, refer to your employment agreement for clarity. If the agreement does not address ownership explicitly, implicit ownership most likely accrues to the academic institution or corporation.

5. **In today's litigious society, people often believe that their status as employees offers protection from legal action.** Those lawyers you think will protect you are paid by your employer, not by you, and that is where they will focus in times of legal assault. Even if you have some level of legal protection through insurance, and even if you're "in the right," you might not be able to survive being right. Lawsuits, even frivolous ones, can last a decade or more. The litigant with the deepest pockets usually prevails because "he who has the gold rules." The ability to outlast the other side is often the determining factor in legal matters.

6. **Knowing when to stay in and when to give in has to be the most difficult decision that presents itself.** So much emotion surrounds this scenario. Often, the decision centers on staying in an organization or leaving it. No matter what the circumstances, you must understand the cost of staying where you are doing what you are doing (both now and in the future). In this instance, opportunity costs come into

play again. If you cannot separate the emotion from the decision, seek professional counsel to help you sort it all out.

7. **Understand how the meaning of *partnership* differs from the practice of it.** Perhaps you and your best friend agree to work together to start a business. You'll make sure to keep your new responsibilities unrelated to your current role in nursing, of course, but you need still to take the time to write down who owns how much of the business, the worth of that ownership, what happens to it if someone wants to walk away, and your respective roles and responsibilities. You'll be glad you did (whether you stay in the business or not).

8. **Realize that no such thing as a new business model exists.** All businesses operate to make money. What sets the business apart is how the business manages and disposes of its money. At this point, nurse executives hit the ceiling when aligning their skills with entrepreneurship from the point-of-revenue production. Historically, our profession evolved from costs. A quick lesson in revenue production: Costing, pricing, billing, and charging for services each represent different points in making money. What a system costs you in dollars and cents does not equate to the price you charge for that service. You need to add a percentage of profit that is market competitive and evolutionary enough to prepare you for the future research and development necessary to keep your product competitive in the marketplace. You must present a bill to your customer for your services or product. They might not actually pay that amount, though, perhaps because you have a percentage discount agreement (a larger contract covering costs for the services that decreases cost

and increases volume). You don't get the money you expected to cover your cost, so how do you make it up? In volume? Through decreased scope of services? While appearing to be a simple calculation, the pricing decision often holds the key to the company's long-term survival.

One of the advantages of intrapreneuring is those hidden dollars that you don't think about with your current employer. When individuals don't quote you a full year's economic value, including benefits, you do not have a picture of that person's total income. You never see on your paycheck the dollars that your employer pays above and beyond the paycheck you receive. From vacation days paid to holidays paid, there are nonproductive hours of pay that you now assume into the costs of operating your business. The employer contribution to employees' Social Security costs, the expense of health care, disability worker's compensation insurance; and myriad taxes paid to states, the federal government, and local cities and towns.

The fact that you are new to operating a business does not entitle you to any break from the law. Ignorance of the law or lack of knowledge aside, you are still responsible for every decision. Don't jump into business ownership until you understand the risks and are ready.

9. **Understand how the organization's overarching relationships and contractual agreements affect you.** You may be employed "at will," but these relationships and agreements exert tremendous pressure over your employment, especially in these days of widespread consolidation.

10. **You *must* take more than a passing interest in the financial health of the organization that owns your facility.** If you think that the practice of

nursing happens far away from these monolithic corporations, you are mistaken. Today, you can find out online how much the top five executives in your corporate organization make, nonprofit and for-profit alike. Don't negotiate your compensation package without knowing all the facts.

Whether nurses thrive inside the organizations where they currently work, seek out a new nursing environment, or leave health care altogether, they must chart a course to their own satisfaction. The course differs for each nurse, which means that the chance to actively engage in reinvention will likely present itself to you several times. Will you choose to reengage where you are, remain the same, move on, or go outside? Whereas the good news is that the choice is up to you, there is even better news: No matter what you decide, you can always decide again.

MEN IN NURSING BUSINESS WORLD SURVIVAL TIPS

Protect yourself legally; the organization won't.

Weigh all your options, short-term and long-term, inside and outside the corporation, as you decide whether to stay or go.

If you go out on your own, you'll be paying all those taxes, insurance premiums, retirement matches, and other benefits the corporation now pays for you.

Remember to calculate the most important expense of all—lost opportunity cost. Whether you stay or go, there are lost opportunity costs associated with each option.

If you decide to make the leap to go out on your own, be smart and assemble an informal board of directors or "kitchen cabinet" to prevent you from drinking your own bath water.

No decision is ever final—you can always decide again.

References

Gerber, M. (1995). *The e-myth revisited: Why most small businesses don't work and what to do about it.* New York, NY: HarperCollins.

Pinchot, G. (1985). *Intrapreneuring: Why you don't have to leave the corporation to become an entrepreneur.* San Francisco, CA: Berrett-Koehler Publishers.

Pinchot, G. (2011). The intrapreneur's ten commandments—The Pinchot perspective. Retrieved from http://www.pinchot. com/2011/11/the-intrapreneurs-ten-commandments.html

Chapter 12
A Male Student's Survival Guide for Nursing School

Spencer Barrington Stubbs
University of Pennsylvania

I remember the words "Hoorah! Hoorah! Penn-syl-va-ni-a!" loudly printed in spirited red and blue ink on my acceptance letter to the University of Pennsylvania back in the spring of 2009 like it was yesterday. I remember proudly standing in front of my mirror trying on my scrubs before my first clinical rotation at the Living Independently For Elders (LIFE) center in West Philadelphia. I remember my successes and my failures; but, most of all, I remember how my time at Penn as a nursing student has felt overwhelmingly difficult at times due to the sole fact that I am a man. That's right—based on my gender. In any other context, this would not be the truth; in nursing school, though, men are the overwhelming minority and can at times suffer from it. And even though I have heard conflicting messages, both explicitly and implicitly, about my belonging in this profession, I have quickly learned to hold on tight to Gary Veale's, BSN, RN, message of "whether a person is a male or female, a nurse is a nurse." I am inspired to write this chapter because I believe it is important for men seeking entry into and, most important, completing a bachelor of science in nursing (BSN) degree to be well equipped with the knowledge needed to anticipate the many potholes that exist along this long and arduous road. Yes, it's a lot to condense into one chapter, but I will do my best to outline a few of the tips that I have used to find success during my time in nursing school.

Tip 1: Find the Right Clinical Instructor

To put it bluntly, your clinical instructor can make or break your clinical experience. All nursing students find this out at some point or another in their clinical experience. Ideally, though, you want to find this out sooner rather than later because the coursework only gets harder as you progress along the curriculum. If you are reading this and know that you have passed the deadline to change your instructor, stay calm, take a deep breath, and make the best of it. If you can still switch, though, do it. Do it, and do not look back.

Like Penn, many schools have valuable online resources that students can access to look at the ratings for each of the clinical instructors. I personally made it a priority to do this not only for each of my clinical courses but also for all of my classes that I take at Penn. Keep in mind, however, that such a small sample size can skew these ratings a little. At Penn, many clinical sections do not exceed eight or nine students, so you have to closely scrutinize a score of 2.0, for example, out of 4.0, if only five students rate this one clinical instructor. Then again, you can investigate a bit to put this 2.0 into better context. More specifically, you should do two things:

1. Look at the clinical instructor's ratings from the other semesters and compare it to the 2.0 (or whatever the score is) that he/she received now.

2. Ask other nursing students what they have heard about your instructor.

Essentially, you want to determine whether this clinical instructor is a one-time offender or is a recurrent bad apple consistently proven to be a thorn in many nursing students' sides.

Of course, having the right clinical instructor constitutes a more general tip that all nursing students (and college students in general, really) can benefit from. Still, in some instances, like the one I'm about to outline, it's particularly crucial for male nursing students to pick the best (and most supportive) clinical instructor possible.

A great deal of research shows the continual marginalization of male nursing students in their obstetrics/labor & delivery (L&D) clinical rotations (Bush, 1976; O'Lynn, 2004). As a male, you will understandably feel nervous about this clinical rotation. Based on your gender, it is sometimes more difficult for you to thrive in certain specialties (for example, women's health) than others. One time on the L&D unit, the attending physician on duty did not want me or the other male nurse in my group to work with his patients. In another instance, I was trying to educate the mother on how to properly hold her baby so that it could latch on to her breasts correctly for proper feeding. I remember how awkward she seemed after learning how to properly hold her baby because she didn't want to demonstrate her newly learned skill in front of me. As a result, she indirectly projected her anxiety onto me and made me just as nervous. One friend of mine even had an instructor who only let the girls in the clinical group into the delivery room.

If you face any of these situations, do not panic. Open up and maintain a steady stream of communication between you and the clinicians and the patients under your care. Introduce yourself as a student and express that you have come to that unit to learn, first and foremost, so seeing and doing as much as possible while on the unit is of the utmost importance. And, yes, this means performing a proper breast and pelvic examination to ensure that your patient maintains proper antenatal care.

So before you are forced to be in a defensive "survival" situation in your clinical, be wise and put some effort into searching for a great clinical instructor; after all, they are the ones who will ensure that you have the best experience possible. Having someone like the clinical instructor on your side when you are on an L&D unit can prove beneficial because he or she holds a certain level of professional clout. For example, I was fortunate to have an excellent instructor during my L&D rotation. She came into the room with me and acted as a buffer between the patient and me so as to make sure that we both felt comfortable and that, most important, I got to see and do as much as possible. So, because finding the right clinical instructor can make or break your clinical experience, choose wisely.

Tip 2: Find a Male Role Model

The typical male nursing student may have few male role models who are currently in the profession. This is crucial because mentors serve as your examples of behavior in clinical settings, professionalism, and, of course, scholarly excellence. And although both men and women in this field can be excellent clinical mentors, as a male nursing student in a female-dominated profession, you should cling to your male role models because some of you might not feel comfortable discussing some issues with a female colleague. Female nurses may be unaware of the subtle discriminatory practices, and slight privilege if you will, that a more seasoned male nurse has experienced and can detect more readily.

My own experience in clinical inspired this tip to a certain extent, but an even greater inspiration for it derives from something one of my closest friends (Frank, a male nursing student in a southern nursing school) told me a few months before I began writing this chapter.

FRANK'S STORY

Frank has always been a hardworking student, to say the least. Because of this effort, he excelled freshman year in all of his theoretical coursework (biology, chemistry, human development, and so on). For the most part, the number of hours he put into his studies reflected the grade he received. Not until the start of his sophomore year, when the school's curriculum started to introduce clinical coursework into the sequence, did Frank realize that he had trouble with the more applied science courses. In fact, he struggled through his first clinical course in the fall and was halfway through his second clinical course in the spring before the course director approached him on the eve of his last exam. She reminded him that if he did not pass the last exam he would fail the course and would have to repeat it the following spring.

Frank, obviously in a state of panic and dismay, went to the first person he could think of for advice: a male nursing professor whom he met freshman year during student orientation. Even though it was last minute, the professor made Frank stay in his office for the rest of the day so that they could go through each of the lectures covered on his last exam. Because Frank struggled with these applied science courses, the professor then took Frank to the lab, way past hours, so that he could practice doing a full head-to-toe physical assessment, taking vitals, reconstituting medications, and so on. Although it took hours to complete, the payoff proved well worth it because Frank not only passed the course but also gained a newfound mentor. After Frank passed the exam, the professor looked him straight in the eyes and told him, "Don't you ever wait until the last minute to seek my help again, do you understand? We'll work together to see you through this program from start to finish—mark my words. We need more male nurses!"

It is your responsibility to be proactive, just like Frank, and to find a male mentor who you can connect with. This male figure can provide you with the advice, insight, and familiarity that a female figure would be less likely able to give. You can start by looking at the list of professors/instructors on your school's intranet/database. Look for common interests and start from there. Also, look to see whether the potential mentor is working on any research/clinical projects and needs assistance; this is a great way to establish and maintain a professional relationship that could potentially flourish into a more personally rewarding one.

Tip 3: Find a Male Nursing Student Network

One of the most powerful things you can do as a student is to build a rapport with other like-minded students while you are in college. You can do so in many different ways, but the easiest is to get involved with a student organization on campus and use this group as a platform to strengthen your bonds with other students. As a male nursing student, you are a clear minority among your peers, so get involved with a group dedicated to serving minorities in nursing, males in nursing, or the like. At the University of Pennsylvania, for example, a group called the Male Association of Nursing (MAN-UP) seeks to serve as a support system for male nursing students on campus. The organization welcomes all members of the Penn community as well as members of the surrounding area interested in issues related to men in the nursing field and men's health. As the group's president, I'm charged with upholding the following tenets for our charter:

1. Provide a forum for discussion of factors affecting male nurses and men interested in pursuing a career in nursing.

2. Act as a collective voice to speak out in support of men in nursing and bring to light inadequacies in nursing education and nursing practice.

3. Assist in recruiting and retaining male nursing students (including but certainly not limited to high school outreach).

4. Organize school- and campus-wide educational opportunities on men's health promotion.

5. Support members academically, socially, and professionally.

6. Foster a spirit of collaboration with national nursing organizations.

7. Provide community service opportunities.

Above all, MAN-UP and other similar organizations provide you, the male nursing student, with not only a strong professional and academic network but also a family. Meetings serve as safe spaces to vent about any frustrations you might have about the curriculum in general and about how you feel treated inside and outside of the classroom/clinical space specifically.

NOTE

One close friend of mine who goes to a nursing school in Philadelphia describes the student group that serves male students in a similar fashion to MAN-UP as a "safe haven." He recalled to me that one time in his freshman year everyone was freaking out about an anatomy and physiology final but that all the male nurses in the group pulled together a succinct study guide and exchanged notes via their group's listserv. He said, "Even though it was during the most academically stressful times in my life, it was pretty inspiring to see a group of male nurses come together and work to see all of us succeed. That could only happen in this group."

Besides basic exam help and notes sharing, group listservs like MAN-UP and others offer professional and postgraduate linkages as well. Many different types of information circulate among group members, including information about internships, externships, research possibilities, and postgraduate job prospects. Such listservs may even provide an advantage to the male nurses, giving them some leverage when it comes to these sorts of prospects. So, join a male nursing interest group, whether on campus or elsewhere, so that you can develop this type of extensive network. These types of actions can only enhance your experience in college and help you succeed.

Tip 4: Get Organized and Start Early

Molecules, molecules, molecules! With general chemistry, organic chemistry, and biology, I can confidently say that I have had my fair exposure to everything and anything molecular based. These courses also forewarned how daunting a nursing curriculum can be. It doesn't matter if you are an AP chemistry/biology scholar in high school or even a co-author for the next journal publication for genomic discovery; everyone collectively hits a wall when studying for these intro courses in nursing school. And it makes sense. Think about it: Freshman year is a year of firsts (especially if you're someone such as I who traveled some distance away from home to receive an education). It's your first time living on your own, making your own schedule (no more standardized 8 a.m. to 4 p.m. schooldays), making your own meals, and for many, stepping out of your comfort zone to make your own friends and form your own social circles. So, that first year can be a huge adjustment for students' social lives. This explains why you have these paradoxes where students who theoretically should thrive in these science classes perform poorly because they are letting their newly inundated social issues invade their academics.

So, my first suggestion for nursing school is to keep your feet planted and reel it in. After all, those who successfully make it through the first year of nursing school are those who seek out the resources needed to thrive in their new college environment. Some schools, like Penn, have specific departments/buildings on campus whose sole purpose is to ensure that students stay on track with their assignments.

If your school doesn't have resources, don't stress; you'll just have to get yourself a planner instead and map out all of your assignments/exams for the semester. I even go a little further and have two separate planners: one for academics and the other for extracurricular events. I've seen people do many variations, mapping out their tasks on their phones or through Gmail or through sticky notes that they place around their room. Whatever the method, the intended goal remains the same: Get as organized as possible. Between labs, lectures, homework, patient case studies, clinical modules, and validation, nursing school throws a lot at you academically, and it's your job to sort everything out to make sure that nothing catches you off guard. So, take a deep breath, stay calm, reel in everything and anything that nursing throws at you, and map out all of your academic (and social) responsibilities. Remember, what makes nurses so great at being clinicians charged with the responsibility of maintaining the continuity of care for all their patients is the fact that they are organized and have excellent time-management skills. From the first time that you walk into the classroom, nursing school forces you to develop these time-management skills; you want to hone them early on, too, so that when you are a fully autonomous RN, time management won't present an issue in the clinical setting.

Tip 5: Practice Makes Perfect

The one thing that sets you apart from your peers who may major in the humanities or the social sciences is that nursing is a very pre-professional major. By *pre-professional* I mean that by being a nursing student you forfeit your right to be a normal student.

NOTE

I'm being somewhat facetious when I say that, but honestly you can't do some of the things that your other peers would do while you're in nursing school. You have to maintain a certain level of responsibility, professionalism, and accountability. For one, you can't just miss clinical. At Penn, for example, they teach us that being sick is not a good enough excuse to miss lecture, lab, or, more importantly, clinical. Penn teaches us to uphold a certain level of responsibility and accountability during times of crises like this. They push us to take a further step in action to make sure that we provide proper documentation to support any medical illnesses, call our instructors before clinical (not during or after), and then make arrangements with the course directors to schedule a make-up day. If any one of these actions is not taken, your medical illness is null and void and punitive actions (i.e., clinical fee, point deductions, etc) will be taken. At first it seems harsh but Penn is trying to teach us early on to live up to the mantra of, "To whom much is given, much is expected." After we graduate and we are in the "real world," so to speak, skipping work without taking necessary preventative measures of covering yourself (i.e., calling, sending an email, etc.) will end up in your losing your job. Thus, when all is said and done, nursing schools across the country would be doing their students a disservice if they didn't also incorporate professional skills as well.

Furthermore, professional golfer Severiano "Seve" Ballesteros once said that "to give yourself the best possible chance of playing to your potential, you must prepare for every eventuality. That means practice." Nursing is a science that, like golf, requires a certain skill set needed for success. You can acquire this skill set only through hard work and dedication. Because the major is so hands-on, you can learn only by putting in the extra hours in the lab/clinical practice sessions. It's one thing to be able to read how to reconstitute medications, hang an IV piggyback, or insert a tracheal tube. Clinical nursing represents another thing altogether, though, because you must apply/practice these techniques so that you'll be ready to perform them when you actually work as an RN.

If you get discouraged with all this work, keep calm and realize that the beauty of a major like nursing is that practice definitely makes perfect. Other majors test proficiency only through exams or papers, frustratingly unpredictable methods. Yes, nursing does have a certain level of unpredictability, which makes it exciting, as well, but it also has a certain level of standardization in the form of skill set you can practice. Once you learn and master the skill set, you can easily adapt it to any patient and any scenario.

Yes, nursing has little margin for error because at every minute you are dealing with people's lives. However, if at any point you do not understand a certain skill (taking a blood pressure, auscultation of lung sounds, and so forth), you can get the necessary help from your instructor to learn that skill. The last thing you want to do is just sweep that skill under the rug and convince yourself that you will learn it later. Again, what so differentiates nursing from other fields is that it is a pre-professional major in which everything, in one way or another, builds off something else. Everything will come back to haunt you. It is up to you to be proactive. Make it a point to schedule extra practice hours weekly to review all the skills you have learned up to that point.

> **NOTE**
>
> *At Penn, on top of having a clinical sequence tied to theory/lecture, we also have mandatory lab sessions to practice the skills used in clinical. We also get periodically tested in lab through clinical simulations (mock case scenarios that test all the skills learned up to that point). Nursing students always find these simulations daunting because they are, of course, cumulative and require you to perform at a certain level of mastery in terms of clinical competence. What a lot of students do, and what I particularly recommend for other nursing students as well, is to schedule practice sessions through open labs a couple of weeks before they validate to sharpen their skills needed to succeed.*

It sounds like a no-brainer, but really, practice makes perfect. The ones who succeed in nursing school and go on to become great nurses aren't the ones who ace all the theoretical exams; instead, they're the ones who make it a point to succeed in clinical. To do this, though, they practice!

Tip 6: Keep a Healthy Mind and Spirit

Last, but certainly not least, with a rigorous schedule that involves lack of sleep and standing on your feet for hours on end, it is no surprise that nursing school can challenge any student. One thing that you might not notice through all of this, though, is your mental health. Having a stable and sound mind and spirit is equally as important to ensuring that you are fit enough to perform to the best of your abilities in clinical; in fact, these two factors are not mutually exclusive. You will face many personal/familial issues during your time in nursing school. These personal issues can range from a break up with a long-time partner to a death in the family of someone who was near and dear to you. No matter the issue, any one of them has the potential to cripple you mentally and to encroach on your performance in nursing school.

To put the importance of this in context, suicide is the second leading cause of death among college students. Depression is not just feeling sad. According to statistics compiled at the Screen for Mental Health website, in a 12-month period nearly 1 out of 10 students will report being depressed enough to seriously consider suicide ("Depression," 2010). In addition, men are much less likely to reach out when they feel depressed and are contemplating suicide. When men attempt suicide, we use extremely lethal means to do so such as guns and hanging ("Depression," 2010). This makes depression among men an extremely precarious and volatile condition.

Male nursing students need to take advantage of all of their school's resources if at any time they feel that their personal issues turn into problems inside the classroom/clinical. Penn, for example, has many resources on campus, such as the Counseling and Psychological Services (CAPS) building, which serves to help all students unpack any personal, emotional, or mental issues they might have. Yes, relationships with faculty mentors, friends, and other colleagues are beneficial, but having an unbiased person to talk to will help you (with an outsider-looking-in perspective) to resolve any issues that you may be experiencing. In sum, keep a healthy mind and spirit to get through this daunting program. You owe it to yourself and to your patients.

In almost any other facet of American culture, men are usually the clear majority. However, in nursing, a profession dominated by women, men are the overwhelming minority and therefore at a higher risk of facing institutional discrimination in the clinical setting. This chapter serves as a guide for you as a male nursing student. As a male nursing student myself, I share these tips so that other men can use them to find success in their respective bachelor of science in nursing (BSN) curriculum. Keeping these tips in mind while also holding on to Gary Veale's message of "whether a person is a male or female, a nurse is a nurse" can help you keep your focus and passion set on successfully completing your BSN degree.

MEN IN NURSING SCHOOL SURVIVAL TIPS

Find the right clinical instructor.

Find a male role model.

Find a male nursing student network.

Get organized and start early.

Practice, practice, practice.

Keep a healthy mind and spirit.

References

Bush, P. J. (1976). The male nurse: A challenge to traditional role identities. *Nursing Forum, 15*(4), 390-405.

Depression. (2010). Retrieved from the Screening for Mental Health website at http://www.mentalhealthscreening.org/info-and-facts/depression.aspx

O'Lynn, C. E. (2004). Gender-based barriers for male students in nursing education programs: Prevalence and perceived importance. *Journal of Nursing Education, 43*(5), 223-36.

Index